The Sex Talk:
A Survival Guide for Parents

by

Joanna Hyatt

Yellow Monkey Publishing Los Angeles

Yellow Monkey Publishing
2305 Glendale Blvd, #202
Los Angeles, CA 90039

Printed in the United States of America

Hyatt, Joanna C.
The Sex Talk: A Survival Guide for Parents/ Joanna Hyatt
p. cm.
Includes bibliographical references
ISBN 978-0-9889058-0-1
1. Parenting-Children and Teens-Sexuality. 2. Sex Education-Teens-Parenting Resources

This book is not intended as a substitute for the medical advice of physicians.

Cover design by Bistro Studios.
Editing/Proofreading by Georgia Davis.

This book would not have been possible without a husband who tirelessly supported me through the entire process, my own parents who modeled great parenting, and the thousands of teens and their parents who have helped shape this book with their stories and their questions.

To all of you, thank you.

Contents

The Part of the Book People Skip
(also known as the Introduction)

This book might take you a little time to get through.

Why? Because you're going to have to do some work. Don't give me that face. This is to help you. I'm not satisfied to have you simply nod along at the brilliant things I say and laugh at my awesome jokes, only to finish the book, walk away and apply a mere 2% of what you read.

Think about why you're reading this book in the first place. On some level you realize that you cannot indefinitely put off talking about "it" with your child. And if you're going to go through all this trouble, why not do it well? Doing this requires you to engage with this book, think through the questions I ask, then, roll up your sleeves and get a little dirty.

Confession: when books ask me to think about a question, to complete some sort of activity in order to master a life-changing principal...I skip it. Even though it will probably improve me as a person, make me more efficient, and fast track me to the Presidency, it also requires that I think, change my outlook, my habits, and my *life*. Ugh. So much work. So, I understand if your first inclination might be to skim pages and skip the application questions.

However, in this instance, your business won't fail or your leadership potential flat line because you decided to do that.

This time, it will be your child who loses. That kid down the hall who is trying to navigate the changes in their body, the roller coaster of hormones, and the million voices screaming for their attention and control of their life. They will be the one that gets the raw end of the deal, suffering because you didn't put in the work.

Consider that my "Win One For The Gipper" speech. You can do this. You *need* to do this. Not for you. And certainly not for me. For your kid(s). And for every kid they're going to meet, hang out with, and date.

Three things you need to accept before we get started:

1. You're going to make mistakes, which means you will say things that sound great in your head but come out wrong.

2. Talking about sex with your kids does not guarantee they will enthusiastically embrace what you teach, or award you for being Parent of the Year. Yet under no circumstance should you give up. As someone who does this for a living (awkward talks with the world's most hostile audiences), I can assure you that they really do want to talk about all these issues. Not just with anyone, but with you. Nevertheless, you should still brace yourself for some initial arguing, shouting, slammed doors, shrieks and groans of awkwardness.

3. I don't have all the answers. No one does. But I'm willing to share everything I've learned working with thousands of teens.

On that note.....let's do this!

FIRST THINGS FIRST

A child of five would understand this. Send someone to fetch a child of five.

Groucho Marx

Chapter 1: The Warm-Up

Thanks to Google, Glee, Jersey Shore and Miley Cyrus, today's kids have the basics of sex figured out not long after they kick their training wheels to the curb. Abstinence has become a four-letter word and sexuality something to be 'explored' once the teething process has concluded. In our culture, sleeping around is as commonplace as hitting the gym, and the quick road to fame and success is leaking a sex tape to the general public.

As your child's parent, you have a choice about how you would like these conversations to go, or at least how you would like your end of the talk to go. There's the "Sex will send you to hell. Once you do it, you're damaged goods," approach. Not the most effective option in the box, but one that some prefer. Or there's the more thoughtful, informed, ongoing dialogue approach. Your call.

Personally, I prefer the approach that treats your son or daughter as a smart, curious, and thoughtful human being. Perfect, definitely not. Difficult, absolutely. But your child has questions that need answering, opinions that are worth hearing and the ability to reason beyond their momentary impulse. I see it every day in the teens with whom I work. If you prefer the later approach then we're off to a good start. If you want the Hell, Fire and Damnation route, all I have to say is....good luck with that.

Time for a....Pop Quiz!

Question #1: In the United States, how many people will contract a new Sexually Transmitted Diseases (STD) this year?

A. 3 million
B. 19 million
C. 37 million

For those of you who picked B, Johnny, tell them what they've won!

This year, nineteen million people will contract an STD in the United States. That is more than the population of America's four largest cities, combined.* It's also a whole lot of people walking around with something gross in

* New York, Los Angeles, Chicago and Houston.

their pants, many of which don't even know it! Nearly half are young people between the ages of 15 to 25 years old, and if my calculations are correct, it means that as a parent reading this book, you have at least one child smack in the middle of the most at-risk group for an STD in America. Or you'll have one there very shortly. This same age group is also the most at-risk for getting HIV, of any group that is sexually active.[1] I'm talking about the United States. Not Africa. Not the brothels of Thailand. Here.

Later on I'll cover the Fab Four of STDs that you should know and be able to discuss with your child. For now it is enough to remember that your child faces a higher risk for getting an STD than you did at their age. And, these STDs have grown bigger and uglier. Times are a changin' my friend.

Question #2: The right time to begin having conversations about sex, dating and relationships is when your child:

A. Approaches puberty
B. Begins High School
C. Goes on their first date
D. Moves out of your house, away from your watchful eye

Correct Answer: A

Those of you with younger children (nine or ten year olds) may think that there is still plenty of time before the onset of puberty forces this conversation on you. With at least a couple of years to go before all hell breaks loose, you're patting yourself on the back for being so ahead of the game in reading this book.

Not to rain on your parade, but a study published in January of 2010 looked at the timing of parents talking to their children about sexuality relative to the child's sexual behaviors. Translation: when did mom and dad finally start talking to their kids compared to when their kids actually started to be sexually active? You might assume the parents got a few conversations in before the kids started to do anything. But we know what assuming does...

This study found that over half of kids engage in genital touching and oral sex before having any discussions with their parents about birth control or condoms, how to resist partner pressure for sex, sexually transmitted diseases and symptoms. Over forty percent of young people have intercourse before any discussion about sexually transmitted disease symptoms, condom use, choosing birth control, or what to do if their partner refuses to wear a condom.[2]

Read that again. Over HALF of children will engage in genital touching and oral sex before their parents even have a chance to talk to them. Of kids that have sexual intercourse, nearly half of them will do so without first having a chat with mom or dad about what is at risk physically and emotionally. Most of the parents of these kids probably plan to have a talk at some point but are afraid of doing so too early. After all, how much can your little 11 year old actually know about all this?

Probably more than you did at eleven. And definitely more than you think. The reality is that for most of us, we're actually not starting to talk with them early enough. I will spare you the stories I read of 5th graders having sex (or attempting to), kindergartners caught in the coat closet fondling each other and 13 yr olds getting pregnant.

This is not just happening in Los Angeles or New York, those presumably heathen cesspools of immorality. Whether your children are in the trendiest urban city or a quiet cow town, they are growing up in a world that is changing at an alarming rate. With cell phones, wireless internet, blatant displays of soft core pornography on billboards and in commercials and sexuality brazenly discussed on radio stations, the covers of magazines and among teens on Facebook, Formspring, or Twitter, it is hard to find a corner of this country that has not been invaded in some way by this sexually permissive culture. Your child is seeing and hearing about sex at an earlier age than you might expect. Even if you were to rigorously monitor TV shows and reading material, friends may be more than enough of an influence to push a teen towards sexual activity.

Question #3: True or False

1. Your child can get an STD from sitting on a toilet seat
2. Oral sex is safer than vaginal sex
3. Anal sex poses minimal health risks because STDs cannot be transferred to the anus
4. Heavy kissing offers no risk for getting an STD
5. Genital skin-to-skin contact is the safest form of sexual activity as there is no penetration or exchange of fluids.

Finished answering? If you picked False for all five questions, then you would be correct. Let me break it down.

1. **Toilet Seat:** While there is probably a .00001% chance that someone could get an infection from a toilet seat, they'd really have to rub themselves all over it.* This is often a common misconception among teens, so make sure you clear that up. Please still encourage the use of toilet seat covers in public restrooms. How many thousands of other naked rear ends have sat on that thing, bringing in who knows what?

2. **Oral Sex:** Oral sex poses just as high of a risk as vaginal sex for being able to contract or pass along an STD. It may be a way to avoid pregnancy, but bacteria and viruses are still transferrable to a person's mouth from another person's genitals or vice versa. There have been reported cases of Chlamydia in the throat, Gonorrhea in the eye, and even outbreaks in the ear. But I digress. A recent report published by Ohio University found that sixty percent of throat and neck cancers were caused by HPV, not tobacco. Which means that oral sex is now riskier than smoking for your child.[3]

The preferred alternative to vaginal sex for those teens wanting to avoid sexual intercourse is now posing its own serious risks. In teen vernacular, oral sex is known as a blow-job, going down on someone or eating out.

---

* That is not a statistical number. I made it up to make a point.

Don't look at me! I didn't come up with the words. I'm just helping you to be in the know.

3. **Anal Sex:** Like oral sex, anal sex is also a high-risk activity for contracting an STI, such as HIV or HPV (see below in my "Fab Four" List). Anal sex also poses serious health risks to the body because it can cause microscopic cuts along the anus, opening a person up for further infection directly into their system. It's not like everything coming out of there is Purel Hand Sanitizer. Not to mention that repeated anal sex can cause colon and rectum issues. Moving on...

4. **Heavy Kissing:** There is minimal risk here, especially if blood is exchanged. If someone has an open sore or cut in their mouth, then their partner could be exposed to whatever they've got, particularly if the sore is Syphilis, a highly contagious bacteria. Even then, you would still have to be swapping buckets of spit or digest someone's blood from a cut in order to contract the infection. I would hope your child is not so desperate for a kiss that they'll still go at it when there is an open sore or blood oozing out. This isn't *Twilight.* No need to suck blood to show love.

5. **Genital skin-to-skin contact:** Probably the one on the list that parents and teens most discount. After

all, how could you possible catch anything just from rubbing your (naked) body up against someone? Don't you at least have to have some sort of fluid exchange? Nope. These little creepy crawlers just need to come in contact with a warm body in order to open shop. Genital herpes sheds on to another person and the Syphilis bacteria can bore into a body wherever it comes in contact. So, if your son or daughter is simply taking their clothes off and making-out (a short hop to further sexual activity), they are still very much at risk.[4]

Question #4: How many teenagers in the United States will become pregnant this year?

A. 100,000-300,000
B. 300,001-550,000
C. Over 550,000

The answer you're looking for is C. Every year, 750,000 teenagers will become pregnant in the United States. All of them girls. But they didn't get there by themselves. Teen and young adult men are also impacted, as are their families. At least the families that know their teen is or was pregnant, or got someone pregnant.

Last question. You're doing great! Or maybe you're failing this abysmally, but I'm proud of you for sticking with me. That alone gets you a gold star.

Question #5: If used consistently and correctly, a condom is how effective in protecting against Chlamydia, Gonorrhea and Syphilis?

A. 98%
B. 85%
C. 50%
D. Only as far as you can throw it.

You picked D, right? Just kidding. The correct answer here is C, 50%.[5] Yes, you read that correctly. Five-O. One out of two. Half of the time. It doesn't matter what or how you name it, a person is still at risk for these infections about one out of every two times they engage in sexual activity, *if* they're using a condom correctly every time. The risk is reduced but it is certainly not completely removed. Sorry if that dampened your enthusiasm a bit for these latex mittens.

So how did you do?? Did you pass with flying colors or did you realize there might be a thing or two you could still learn when it comes to talking to your kids about sex and relationships? Whatever your results, by the end of this book, you're going to be a Jedi when it comes to talking about sex and relationships with your teen. Light saber not included.

Chapter 2: Finding the BEST Person to Talk with Your Child

Talking about sex.

Top five on every parent's list of things they enjoy doing with their awkward, pimply-faced teen. Right up there with Chinese water torture and toothpicks shoved under fingernails. Yes, it's just that fun.

Although sex is talked about openly and ad nauseam in our culture, it is still THE taboo topic of conversation between parents and their kids.* The media talks about the sex lives of movie stars, politicians, and athletes. Teens gather in school hallways to talk about what they did last night or during that party last weekend. You talk about it with your married friends and single friends.

* To the person about to give me a schooling in how we're in fact so very repressed, hung up as a society, that we should be more like the Dutch, etc...save it. I can't actually hear you. But you're welcome to email me and we can have a lovely chat.

Siblings even discuss it! But when it comes to parent/teen conversations on sex...everyone clams up.

Why?

Perhaps you're afraid you'll say the wrong thing and do more damage than you would by not saying anything at all. Maybe it's because you don't want to even acknowledge your teen will one day have sex, or could be doing so right now (have you checked on them lately?). It's weird on both sides of the conversation to think that either parent or teen has had sex, will have sex, or even wants sex. It's so intimate....and yet talked about, insinuated about, and joked about. Not to mention thought about by 99% of us.

Recently, I grabbed coffee with a couple and their twin 15-year-old daughters. I was under the impression this was a casual family catch up, with maybe a question or two tossed my way to pointedly talk about teenage relationships (a strategic way for the parents to bring this up around their girls). Strategic it was, but not at all what I expected. After we got our drinks, the father pointed to the twins and me, then to a table with only three chairs and said, "Ok, I'm not going to ask what is discussed or ask any questions. So go ahead and talk about, you know, ah, Joanna, I bought your coffee so you owe me." WHAT?! Really?? That's how you're going to tee up a sex talk between your kids and a woman they barely know? I would have at least preferred a shot of really good scotch instead of the watery drip I was holding. I had no idea where I was supposed to go with this or how much (or little) the parents wanted me to share. Needless to say the following seven minutes were rather awkward. What I did deduce between nervous giggles and averted eye contact was that their parents had never talked to them about sex and the girls were in two very different places , emotionally and relationally.

With so much at stake here – your child's future, health, and overall emotional and relational well-being – it makes sense that you want to get the most qualified person possible to handle this delicate yet critical topic. Even if this requires staging a hijacking like that dad.

You get a plumber to fix your drains (or to fix your failed attempt), so why not get a ... Sex Expert? Sexpert? Is there such a thing? Actually, yes, there is. And in this economy, their rate is actually very reasonable for what you get. All the information you need to contact this person is on the next page. Are you ready for this? Get some pen, some paper! Grab your phone! Everything is about to get so much easier!

INSERT YOUR OWN
PICTURE HERE

You were hoping my cell number was waiting for you, weren't you? While I am here to help and be a resource, an aide, that person to answer the three am call, I'm ultimately not your gal. You want the most effective person you can find and that is...yes, you.

YOU are the greatest influence in your teen's life when it comes to their decisions about sex and relationships.

Don't believe me? You don't have to take my word for it. Here's what teens themselves had to say only after repeated promises that their identity would not be disclosed to their parents:

8 in 10 Number of teens who say it would be easier to avoid early sexual activity and teen pregnancy if they were able to have more open, honest conversations about these topics with their parents.[6]

59: Percent of teens who consider their parents to be role models of healthy, responsible relationships.[7]

Over half of young adolescents (aged 12-14) say parents most influence their decisions about sex.

24: Percent of teens who cite friends as most influential.[8]

There are a lot of voices vying for your child's attention, but they say YOURS is the voice that stands out. What you say on sex and relationships pierces through the cacophony of noise to leave an impression. It would be a strict breech of the Teenage Code of Behavior to say that to your face, but study after study consistently shows them admitting this.

Do you realize what this means? You've just received critical intelligence that your messages *can* and *do* get through enemy lines. How excited are you?? This changes everything. Since this was the only thing holding you back – fear of wasting your breath – you can now speak freely knowing they will be listening with rapt attention (even through those headphones blasting Ke$ha into their brains). Best of luck. Cannot WAIT to get emails of cute anecdotal success stories.

Chapter 3: The Conscientious Objector

You're still here.

So that bit of good news didn't open the floodgates of conversation?

You're not alone. Like most parents, you know that your child's decision to engage (or not engage) in sexual activity could have long-term implications on their life. But you have your reasons for resisting. Perhaps you're paralyzed by your own past, skeptical that all this will backfire on you, or unconvinced that the best person to really do this is you.

Before we go any further, let's address some of the most common objections I hear from parents.

1. "If I Start Talking *About* Sex, Then They May Go *Have* Sex."

Right. Because until YOU planted the seed in their mind, your child had never and would never have thought about sex? I guarantee you they have thought about it, even if it's just idle curiosity. And they have questions, lots of them. But unless you first initiate conversation, there is a slim chance your child will proactively broach the subject. It is up to you to make it clear that this is a topic definitely on the table, and can be brought up at any time.

Even if your teenager is not having sex, if they are hanging out with a great crowd of kids who are making good life choices, or they are living in a cave somewhere high in the mountains, you are still not off the hook.

This is not about getting your kid to avoid a certain behavior. It's about helping them to gain a healthy perspective, to learn to balance their sexuality as part, but not all, of who they are and to equip them to make informed choices they can live with.

2. "Not My Child"

Some of you are rolling your eyes right now, scoffing at the *very idea* that this would ever apply to your child. Let's stay in that state of denial for one moment and consider the kids that your child is friends with, the teens and young adults they are dating, will date, and someday, the man or woman they will marry. Who is teaching *them*?

Maybe your kid isn't going to have sex....and maybe they will. Much of that depends on who they spend time with, whether or not you have taught them how to say no, how to proactively help their friends make healthy choices and most importantly, if they have owned the decision and have a clear understanding of WHY they should postpone sex.

Why NOT your kid, by the way?

Because of your socio economic status? Because they're "smarter" than that? Because of your religion? Because you made vague death threats that if they so much as think about sex, you will take them out of this world as easily as you brought them in to it? Please. You've forgotten then, what it's like to be a teenager battling between the sane and the hormone-crazed sides of your brain, where everything your parents tell you NOT to do instantly jumps to the top of your To Do list.

The last and most common objection:

3. "My past isn't exactly stellar in this area."
As parents, we have all made mistakes. Some are hilarious stories to retell with old friends, others you hope stay hidden deep within the pages of your sparkly

journals. Aren't you glad there weren't Facebook, Twitter, YouTube, and camera phones to immortalize your teenage stupidity?

I was speaking to a group of parents and the above objection came up. As usual, there were some very diverse opinions on how to handle this. One mom was adamant about not telling her teens anything, wanting them to see her as perfect, the shining example of how to make all the right choices. She was even willing to flat out lie if they ever asked her directly. Another parent was of the full disclosure camp, believing that the gritty details would scare the kid out of making the same choices. I think both approaches have noble intentions, but miss the mark.

You're their role model, their hero (even if at times they treat you like the greatest social blight in their life), and the one that is supposed to be showing them how to make good choices. Glibly share too much and you risk proving that a few poor decisions don't have any long-term impact. Zip your lip and you risk your child making the very mistakes you had hoped they would avoid. Lie about your past in an effort to create a 'better' example and you risk losing all credibility once they find out the truth. Any trust you built up, any open doors for communication, are wiped out because they now see that you have been lying to them. If you've been fabricating your past to appear to be something you are not, then how can they trust anything else you say? And don't think they won't find out, at least in part.

It's a fine line my friend, a razor sharp edge upon which you must walk.

I do believe that you should share your past, as it makes you more relatable and gives your words the weight of personal experience. Nothing is as powerful as saying, "I know what you're going through because I've been there myself." Your children may forget from time to time you too were once a teenager (something you're all too happy to forget yourself), struggling with the same temptations, the same hormones, and the same desire to declare your independence. By sharing what you have been through, you are relatable, which is relational gold when dealing with anyone born after 1997. The world is rapidly changing but teenage angst is still very much the same, perhaps just a bit more compounded. You go from the Grinch with a shriveled heart to someone who *knows* the potential consequences because you've experienced them first hand.

How

Your attitude as you broach this with your kids is critical, particularly if your past sexual choices are not what you would want for your own children. You wanting more for your child, wanting different life experiences than you had, does not make you a bad parent. Neither are you a hypocrite for promoting better decisions than those you made. It makes you a parent who loves their child enough to admit that, as a parent, you are not perfect but want more for them.

Don't you do this in other areas? Perhaps you didn't do well in school, or you wish you had gone to college, or you quit a job that you should have stayed with, or dabbled in drugs or [insert your own teen/young adult mistake]. Do you shrug your shoulders and decide it's too much to encourage your kid to make different choices? Not at all. That's why kids *need* parents, to be able to guide them, to help direct them towards a better life and better choices than they themselves made. Again, it's about your attitude.

If you're afraid to share your past, try starting the conversation with something along these lines, "I have not set a good standard for you and I'm about to talk to you about something I myself have failed in. I'm coming to you in humility."

Please, please, do not share the nitty gritty details of your past partners, what you did, how terrible or great it was. No one wants to know that mom was swinging from the chandelier with some guy other than dad. Actually, no one wants to know that, period, even if it was dad. There are limits to what kids need or even should know about their parents. But feel free to talk about *why* you did it (I thought it would make me popular, my friends were pressuring me, I thought he would stay with me, and all other sorts of cliché but tragically true reasons) and how you felt afterward, both in the short term and the long run (I felt taken advantage of, I regretted it, it made it much harder when I married your mom/dad, the memories wouldn't go away, etc).

They may think that you've turned out just fine, that you never had any pain or heartache as a result of your decisions but you have an opportunity to offer them something priceless, something they cannot get on their own: perspective. Hindsight is always 20/20, right? Use that perspective, however painful or mundane it may be, to help explain why you're encouraging them to wait until they're in a committed relationship such as marriage to be sexually active, why you insist on talking about this, and why you're willing to share part of your past with them, even if you're not proud of it.

How many of you wish your parents had done a better job of speaking to you about sex, had been more open about what they learned and at least tried to impart some modicum of wisdom? Don't make the same mistake with your own son or daughter (because maybe if someone had talked to you, things would have turned out differently).

When?

Only you know when it will be appropriate to share, and what will help the conversation and your teen. I say teen because telling your ten year old that you had sex with other people before your spouse might not be the best decision. Doing so when they're 15 years old, believe they're in love (they're not), and struggling to decide whether it is worth it to wait is a different story. They are more mature, have realized by now that you're not perfect (what??) and are themselves facing a big life decision. Sharing your story does not guarantee they won't have sex but it does give them a personal perspective from which to look at this issue. You've taken it from the abstract ("Did you know that 19 million people will get an STD this year?") to a level that they can relate with, because it's you and you've actually lived it.

Not having any 'stories' is also a story! It can be just as effective to relate the good choices you made, when you were glad you did what you did, why it was worth it to wait. There's always an audible gasp when I share that the first time I ever had sex was on my wedding night. "But Ms. Hyatt, *no one* waits anymore." All of our stories matter, whatever they may be. We need to share them with humility and understanding, acknowledging that while what we have faced may not be shared by others, our choices can still encourage, inspire, challenge, and caution others.

Teens need to see every perspective in order to make an informed choice for themselves, not one made out of pressure or desperation. We are shaped by our experiences, but we're also able to help others by them, so don't be afraid to talk with your teens about what you did at their age. You'll be acknowledging that the struggles, feelings and temptations they face are a normal part of life, but they are not the whole of life. Teens own their decisions, their decisions do not own them.

Whatever your past, do not let it hold you back from speaking to your children about these issues. Do not allow it to keep you from painting a picture of what the best scenario could be for your children, or what you believe they are capable of achieving. They have something you may not have had: You.

A parent willing to engage honestly on these critical issues will make more of an impact than any of the thousands of voices screaming at them from the radio, TV, magazines and even their friends. Sadly, parents themselves are having trouble believing this.

Contrast what teens said earlier about parent influence with the following stats from adults themselves:

48 Percent of adults say friends are most influential in their teens decisions about sex.

32 Percent of parents believe they most influence their child's decision about sex[9]

When did we lose confidence in our ability, as parents, to raise our own children? When did we begin to allow other people, companies, ad agencies, news stations, and organizations to be the dominant voice in our teen's life on issues of morality, values, and identity? Yes, the culture has become more sexualized, more aggressive in its promotion of sexuality and sexual behavior. And yes, it is much harder for your teens to avoid sexual activity than ever before. But it is not unrealistic or impossible.

I believe a large reason for the increase among teens in sexual activity, number of partners, pregnancy and STDs is because too many parents have simply stopped engaging their pre-teens and teens on these issues. Or they make a half-hearted attempt, which becomes about as effective as dumping a bucket of water on a blazing forest fire. Rather than ceding the ground on which we stand and laying down our weapons in defeat, we should be all the more driven to fight for our youth, to fight for them to hear the truth, and to fight for them to have an opportunity at a future free from physical and emotional hurt from past sexual choices, and free from broken relationships, depression, and guilt. Fight for them to be free to live life with expectation and hope for what sex could be in a beautiful, loving, intimate committed relationship.

If you stop fighting for your teen, then who will? If you stop making every possible effort to speak into their life, you will leave a gaping, irreplaceable void. You matter. If you have lost confidence in the impact you could make in your child's life, or if your teen has repeatedly told you that your opinion doesn't matter, I am here to say otherwise and to plead with you to engage in this area, and not to lose heart or give up.

If that didn't motivate you, go watch *Braveheart* and then come back. I'll wait.

It's awkward. I get that. If it makes you feel any better, I still get nervous right before speaking to a group of teens, and I actually enjoy doing this. Who knows how they will react to what I have to say? What if it comes out wrong? What if they don't like my outfit and stop listening three seconds in?? But while I get anywhere from a few dozen to a few hundred teens at a time, you have one, two, maybe three teens. Take comfort in knowing that I will never reach those 800 the way you will be able to reach your own child.

Chapter 4: Your Audience

What is the first rule when giving a speech or presentation?

Know Thy Audience.*

Know how they think, their learning style, the way they communicate, what motivates them, excites them and what will make them tune out. You could craft a brilliant, forward thinking speech on social marketing and the rise of new technology, but if it's given to a room full of octogenarians, your words have probably fallen on deaf ears. Literally.

With such an awkward, interesting and simultaneously complex issue as what you're trying to discuss (SEX, in case you forgot), it's critical to know your audience. In this case, your audience is sullen, hormonal, moody, and

* If that's not actually the first rule, oh well. This served my purpose.

confused. They prefer conversations in sound bytes of 140 characters and have no problem refusing to add their own parents as their 'Friend.' The following excerpt from the training manual of Merrill Associates will give you a quick snapshot of what I mean. People have to actually be taught how to deal with Generation Y, the Millenials, aka your kids:

> *Generation Y has never known life without cell phones, pagers, fax machines, and voice mail.*
>
> *Sometimes referred to as the over-achieving, over-scheduled generation, their lives have been programmed from the beginning with school, sports, arts, clubs and activities. They have never known the slow pace of life of their grandparents, when mail was delivered by the Postal Service not the internet. The high tech media driven society of today has opened the world and exposed these young people to more than previous generations even dreamed of.*
>
> *[T]hey are impatient. Life has always moved at a very fast pace. The old adage, "good things come to those who wait," has no meaning for this generation. The internet has taught them there is no need*

to wait for anything - everything is available at the click of a button, from test grades to chat rooms.

For Generation Y the concept of going to the library to find information is foreign. It is instantly available through a Google search. There is no need to look up a movie time in the newspaper, when they can access the information through the wireless web on their cell phone. They have grown up with computers in the classrooms, video games and MTV. They like to be entertained and stimulated across all their sense. Multitasking is part of their routine. They become restless and bored quickly and are constantly looking for the next level of challenge.

The children of "never trust anyone over thirty" parents, this generation has ... watched the confessions of Princess Diana, saw sports figures discredited, and heard a president lie. They have few illusions about what the world is really like and thus are skeptical and wary. They have seen too much to believe everything at face value. Because their skepticism has led them to question much of what they see and hear, they value honesty and truth. They dislike embellishments, half-truths and overinflated promises.

> *Though they often appear disrespectful, they crave respect. They believe that power equals respect. While they are slow to give respect, they expect respect automatically.*
>
> *Finally, they are looking for ways to make their mark and find their causes. When the match is right, they are highly committed and fiercely loyal. [T]hey also expect you to believe in them. They want to be respected, outspoken equals and when they find that "fit" they will be faithful allies.*[10]*

THAT is your audience. Promising, right?? I bet you just can't *wait* to get started after reading that. With such an ADD-multi-tasking-easily bored generation, you have 20 seconds to get their attention. Your child's fast paced, multi-stimulus world means you will need to be intentional about what you say, how you say it and when you say it. It's no longer about having one giant, dreaded "Talk," but instead, lots of little moments that make up an ongoing conversation. This means you have lots of different chances to speak truth into your child's

* I could have come up with my own description, but why do that when I can simply Google, copy, paste and cite? Lazy you say? I like to think of it as efficient. Oh wait, that sounds just like.....yep. I know this generation because I AM this generation. Get excited for the next 160 pages.

world, and dozens of different mediums by which to do so. So be encouraged! If you don't get it right one time, you get a redo the next round.

I don't care how much swagger your son has, or how much attitude your daughter can throw with the flip of her hair. They're insecure, vulnerable, confused and just trying to put up a front while they scramble to figure it all out. Remember when you were a teenager? Yeah, I don't want to either, but we have to in order to relate. Just long enough to remember how rough it really was. I've yet to meet a well-adjusted adult who wishes they could go back to being in high school. Emphasis on well-adjusted. Just because your teens put on an air of independence, arrogance and self-confidence does not mean they are not also struggling with some of the same issues you did. The world may be changing, but how a teen feels has not. If anything, they are MORE confused, MORE insecure, and MORE unsure of who they are and how to act, thanks to this crazy 24/7, all-access world.

Whatever front they put on, if your kids are anything like the thousands of teens I meet each year, they're searching desperately for answers to their questions but having a hard time determining what IS the truth:

What is the truth when it comes to **SEX**?

Is it good or is it bad?

Is it casual, is it sacred?

Is it risky or is it safe?

Is it something to get over with quickly, or to be saved for someone special?

What is the truth when it comes to **RELATIONSHIPS**?

Is dating a thing of the past and hooking up the new path to romantic success?

Is it too forward and traditional to want to actually use titles that denote exclusivity?

Should you be content with a relationship that is more physical than emotional?

What is the truth when it comes to **MARRIAGE**?

Is it even worth it or better just to live together for a while and hope for the best?

What is the point of getting married other than a piece of paper?

Is marriage really as incredible and beautiful as they want to believe it is?

While they're trying to sort out all of these questions, your kids are simultaneously being bombarded with an enormous amount of pressure to conform to what is presented as the 'normal' teenager while being told to express their individuality, to broadcast loud and proud their uniqueness....but only as long as it fits within the approved social script.

Any wonder our teens feel all upside down and inside out?? You would be too if this is what you had to endure every day in a body that has been hijacked by ragging, relentless and uncooperative hormones.

They need you. Not just when they mess up and need to be bailed out. They need you before, during, and after as they wrestle with these big questions and form their own identity. They need to know that they're not "too much," and that you can handle whatever they throw at you.

As you walk down this path with your son or daughter, remember that the person standing in front of you rolling their eyes and slouching into the couch is really just trying to find their way in this world, desperately looking for answers because they actually don't know everything.

Your audience isn't as tough as they seem. They're just very good at pretending otherwise. You have nothing to fear. Except fear itself. And lions and tigers and bears, oh my.

Chapter 5: A Different Perspective

SEX IS GREAT.

What? You didn't see that one coming?

All of you reading this know that's true. How else did you get yourself in this mess of now having to talk to a child about all of this? 'It' can be pretty awesome, but it can also be quite cringe-worthy. It can be hilarious, spicy, awkward, messy, and intimate....all within twenty minutes.

Your opinion about sexual activity has no doubt changed as you have gone through different seasons of your life. As a teen, you may have found it interesting, confusing or been the one handing out tips behind the school bleachers. As you got older and more serious about relationships, it may have become less about pushing boundaries and more about a way to build a connection with someone. Maybe you saw sex as a Molotov cocktail that you didn't dare handle for fear of being scarred for life. Or you were the one trying to hit every person on your campus. You may have been indifferent about the sexual practices of others, or judged everyone who failed to meet the standards of a convent.

Then you had kids.

Sex got a whole lot more complicated, controversial, uncomfortable....and I'm not just talking about between you and your spouse. You joined the ranks of parents who list talking about sex as the most awkward, uncomfortable and dreaded conversation to have with your child. We don't want our kids to hate the very idea of sex, but how do we treat it in a way that won't make it so alluring that they want to run out and do it this very moment? How do you balance the risks-and-consequences talk while still being sex positive? Some of you are slightly terrified at what 'sex positive' even means.

If you knew you would have your child's total attention, and they would remember every word of what you said....what would you want to tell them about sex? What words of wisdom, inspiration, motivation and encouragement would you want to give? What picture would you want to paint for them about what they should be expecting, and the standards they should set. Take some time to think through all of this before you write it down. Don't just give me what you think I want to hear. I'm never going to see this. It's to help *you*. Be sure to write it down so you can refer back to it from time to time. If your child's other parent is involved in their life, these are questions you will want to discuss with them as well as making sure you're on the same page. If you find out they're operating from a completely different book, then you'll at least know what you're up against.*

Jot down your answers right here or on a separate sheet of paper.

1. What do you think about sex?

* You could also use this as a great date night activity! You're welcome.

2. Do you engage in sex when you're "in love"? How do you define love?

3. Do you wait for sex when you are in a committed relationship? What qualifies as committed?

4. Should sex be saved for marriage? Why or why not?

5. What do you think about your child having sex?

6. If you could select the optimum situation for your child to be having sex, what would that be?

Sex has huge implications for your child's life physically, emotionally, and mentally. Sex in the wrong context can be very damaging, immediately and in the long-term. But sex can also be amazing. We are wired to want sex, wired to seek out relationships and intimacy. But sex does not control us. We control it. Too many parents believe that their child's attitude and behavior towards sex is an inevitable part of life over which they, the parents, can have no influence. They brace for the worst and hope for the best. Others see it as a rite of passage, as long as no one gets pregnant or gets a sexually transmitted infection (Especially for sons. Why is that??).

Instead of thinking about sex as:

- The most uncomfortable conversation you will ever have with your teen
- The inevitable teen experience
- A casual encounter with a few people before settling down
- Something so good you need to downplay it, big time, so you're kid will absolutely not find it interesting *at all*

Start thinking about sex as:

- Some of the most meaningful and even fun conversations you will have with your son or daughter
- An educated, and informed choice that your child can make
- In the right context, a rewarding, beautiful and mysterious experience without regrets
- Something to get excited about

Shifting the way we *think* about sex will shift the way we *talk* about sex.

I'd like to let you in on a little secret. I think we're finally at the point in our relationship where we can trust each other.

I WANT YOUNG PEOPLE TO SAVE SEX UNTIL MARRIAGE.

Gasp! Yes, I went there. All the way there. Before you write me off as some Amish fundamentalist, hear me out. It might even give you an idea or two for when you have to answer your own child's "Why?"

I want them to wait because it is the healthiest for them physically and emotionally.

If young people wait until they get married to have sex, there's no risk of an STD. Zilch, none. Unless they marry someone with one of the three viruses that cannot be cured, or a lying cheat. They won't become one of those 19 million who will get an STD this year, or one of the 750,000 annual teen pregnancies. They'll burn deep neurological pathways as they bond with that one person, fostering deep trust, emotional and relational stability and even greater satisfaction than those who do not wait.[11] Even for those who have already been sexually active, choosing to stop and wait will bring the same benefits. As the risk for an STD goes down, their hearts and minds have time to heal.

I want them to wait so that they are free from any haunting memories, any regrets or unnecessary pain.

Not every sexual experience is regrettable, or terrible. But it happens much more than it should. I don't want your child to be the 17 year old girl who came up to me after a talk one day and said, "I've been with my boyfriend for two years and I hate sex. I don't ever want to have it again." Something that should be exciting and happily shared between two people has been broken and distorted for this poor girl. You cannot guarantee your child won't experience this if they have sex without the full promise of the other person's long-term commitment, regardless of what the sex is like at any given time. You cannot guarantee that their fragile psyche and tender teen heart won't be mortally wounded from a sexual experience gone wrong. Kids can be cruel and manipulative. Heck, some adults are that way, but you hope your child will get smarter at reading people as they get older.

I want it because I believe that the decisions young people make today matter in their future marriages, and strong marriages are key to our survival as a society.

I will spare you the sociology lesson on why all that is true. Consider though, when marriages break up or relationships frequently don't even make it to this point, and we begin to have more single parents, moms with children from multiple fathers, children bounced around from home to home because of financial problems and a growing population dependent on government handouts (aka the money their neighbors pay into taxes) rather than being able to support themselves and even contribute in return...don't you think that will begin to have a negative effect on national stability, individual well-being and prosperity and the social fabric as a whole? It doesn't happen overnight. These choices and behaviors are choices that begin as a teenager and develop into habits that become a lifestyle by the time they are well into their adult years. It matters to me that your child starts making it a habit to choose the best, and that they someday enjoy this gloriously difficult thing called marriage.

I want it for them because I have experienced, first hand, how freeing and exhilarating it is to

have waited and then be able to fully enjoy sex in the context of marriage.

Yep, I waited. For a full twenty-five years. I kissed a few guys but there was no oral sex, no getting naked and no hand jobs– even when I was dating the man to whom I'm now married. For twenty-five years, I got first dates, but not many second dates, hung out with my girlfriends *a lot,* and had to explain ad nauseam why in the world I was waiting to have sex. In the moment, it wasn't the easiest or the most exciting, although it often garnered unexpected respect. But it was all worth it.

I don't regret the guys I didn't sleep with. I don't regret that my husband is the only man with whom I'll have memories, that whatever we do is filled with only thoughts of him. Was the honeymoon awkward? Hilariously so, though I will not print the details here because I'm happily married and would like to stay that way. I will say however that I distinctly remember thinking that week how grateful I was that I was experiencing all this with someone who I knew beyond a shadow of a doubt was there for me and not just what I could provide sexually. Someone who wanted to spend the rest of his life figuring out how to get better at sex. With me. I'm having an absolute blast (no, I'm not sexually repressed thank you very much) and want that for every teen and young adult out there.

I want them to wait because sex IS great. And they shouldn't have to settle for anything less.

But we can't paint this terrible horrible picture of all the awful things sex *might* do as a means of scaring them away. It won't go very far in its prevention. Or you'll absolutely terrify them and send them into adulthood with some serious need for therapy.

What if.....

We started talking to teens about sex in such a way that **they start waiting out of expectation for what it *could* be, rather than out of fear for what they could get.**

Take a minute. Let that sink in.

Wouldn't that be a twist to the discussion?

Rather than being the perpetual bearers of bad news, those parents, educators and other adults who encourage sexual integrity in teens would now do so by promoting just how great sex can be within the confines of a committed relationship, such as marriage.*

We raise the bar of expectation by giving our teens and young adults something worth expecting.

The model of sex currently being promoted sells our kids a cheap imitation of the real deal. It treats it as a purely physical act with no real meaning, lasting maybe a few months if couples are lucky, but more often, only a few nights and in the end, what are the two individuals left with? At best, they may have picked up some new moves, learned a thing or two about what not to do next time and if they're lucky, avoided an STD. At worst, they are left physically affected, emotionally unsatisfied, disappointed about failed expectations and trying to ignore the nagging desire for love and commitment that casual sex fails to deliver. Sex is so much more than that!

Definitely educate your kids on the risks of sex outside of a committed relationship, such as marriage, and how to reduce these risks if they choose to be sexually active. Not just the physical impacts but also the emotional.

* In talking about sex differently, let's also replace the word "Abstinence" with "Sexual integrity," and/or "Risk avoidance." Abstinence sounds about as exciting to young people as the words "finals" and "term papers."

Facts, statistics and other information are helpful and useful, which is why you'll be getting plenty of this information in the next few pages. But use that as a contrast to what sex *could* be if they choose to wait, to illustrate *why* you're encouraging them to wait; because you want them to be able to enjoy sex for all that it can be, rather than experience it in a way that may hurt them or leave them disappointed.

Don't be afraid to get them excited about how great sex can be in a committed relationship such as marriage! How freeing it can be when you know you can truly trust that person, the intimacy that comes from knowing the person on a deeper emotional level, and about the communication that is needed for truly great sex. You get the point.

Your shift in attitude is going to change every aspect of your conversations with your kids on these topics. I also find it's much more exciting to be able to talk positively, painting a picture of hope for what could be instead of constantly having to be "Debbie Downer" with stories of gloom and doom.

THE NUTS & BOLTS

Get the facts first, and then you can distort them as much as you please.

Mark Twain

Chapter 6: Back to Basics

I was speaking to a group of 8th grade girls and we were discussing how sexually transmitted infections can effect their sexual organs and reproductive potential. Standard par for the course, when you travel around talking about sex. I quickly realized by the looks on their faces that many of them had not even been schooled on the basics of their body or the changes that puberty would bring, if it had not already. After walking them through what happens during a menstrual cycle, one girl timidly raised her hand and asked, “Is that why we bleed?” Good gracious! How had her mom or dad failed to explain that most basic of female bodily functions? Imagine how frightening, confusing and even embarrassing it must have been for her!

I was terrified when I first got my period, crying to my parents that I didn’t want to grow up (you might say I’m a bit dramatic). My father lovingly told me it was a healthy and normal part of maturing into a woman, (yes, he’s awesome–he once bought tampons for me when I was too embarrassed to do it. World's Best Dad right there) while my mom tried to answer my wailing, "Why???!!!"

How many young teenage boys do not fully understand what an erection is, why they can get one at the slightest breeze, or that 'wet dreams' are a normal part of puberty? For both boys and girls, do they know how to deal with the new found attention from the opposite sex or even people a few years older than they are, as their body changes and matures into the shape of a man or a woman? You need to teach them how to handle all that attention. Unless you're ready to become a grandparent soon.

All of this is basic biology people, and one of the first things to discuss with your child. *Before* they hit puberty. Why then, is this still tripping up parents right out of the gate? Perhaps you think teachers will cover it. Educators can help, but don't completely surrender your child's education to someone else. YOU are the parent. I would kill to have the same degree of influence in your child's life that you do (figure of speech here). While I won't stop trying to encourage, admonish, educate and inspire young people on their sex lives, it will take thousands of my words to do what only dozens of yours will. You are the first and greatest voice in your child's life. Don't give that up. With that privilege, however, comes responsibility. A responsibility to ensure that your child is being taught and raised up knowing the truth: about their bodies, their intrinsic value, how to adjust to the emotional and physical changes of growing-up, and what and when is the best expression of their sexuality. Use other resources and individuals (me, pick me!) to help you know how to maximize this impact.

> *"If I bring attention to their sexual organs, to the changes happening in their body, than they will become curious, confident, begin to experiment and express themselves sexually."*

Are we still there? Your kids are sexual beings. Plain and simple. To deny this only causes harm, both now and later. By not talking about the changes their body undergoes during puberty and the new feelings and sensations they may be experiencing, we may unwittingly create feelings of shame in our children, because if mom and dad refuse to acknowledge it, this must be wrong or abnormal. Or we leave them to explore on their own what these changes mean, without proper guidance and perspective.

The onset of puberty is also an incredible teaching moment to help your child understand how complex and finely tuned their body is, that these changes signal their passage from childhood to adulthood. By being able to educate your child on the amazing transformation they are undergoing, the intricacies of their sexual organs and what this means for their future, you are able to lay a foundation upon which to build a powerful case for postponing sexual activity until a committed relationship, such as marriage. You are teaching them that their body is meant for more than just their own momentary pleasure or as a means for getting what they want. It is a body that is to be protected, cared for, and valued.

Sex is not just sex for an orgasm or because that is what they think all their friends are doing. Sex isn't what you do just to keep a guy from leaving. Sex is about two very unique and complex people coming together to create an emotional and physical bond, to show love in an incredibly powerful way and potentially create life.

Please refrain from using sock puppets or Ken and Barbie to illustrate. And call things by their real name. Shwim-shwam is not a word. Penis. Vagina. Scrotum. Uterus. Say them out loud if you have to in order to get comfortable. Then get out of here and say them to your kid. In a sentence, of course. Just yelling the words on their own will make you sound like you have a strange type of speech impediment. Although it will certainly get their attention.

In speaking about basics, it's imperative that you cover reproduction, baby making, procreation, getting knocked up, how to put a bun in the oven, being preggo....you get the point. You would think this is obvious, especially to your older children, but you might be surprised at the naiveté of some. Or the utter lack of knowledge and blinding sense of invincibility they have.

I had a student send an email to me recently, because she thought she might be pregnant. When I asked how that would be possible (I like to ask teens obvious questions – you'd be surprised what kind of unobvious answers you will get), she replied that it was because she and her boyfriend had been practicing the Potential Parent Method aka "pulling out." And I quote, "I know there is no guarantee but that's what we usually did."

Teens drive fast, jump off bridges, sneak out, go to parties, and practice risky sex because they feel invincible. All those bad statistics, terrible deaths, and teen pregnancies happen to other people. Not them, not ever.

That would just mess up their plans. I'm constantly asking students how many sperm it takes for someone to get pregnant (Just one, by the way, in case there's any confusion). We discuss different ways you can minimize the risk of that one sperm reaching that egg. Or better yet, completely remove the risk until you're ready to be a parent (although let's be honest, how many people are ever really ready when that first one comes? Not me). But if kids grow up thinking a baby comes from swallowing watermelon seeds, the stork, eating play-doh, or sex on just one particular day a month, we're sending them into a minefield.

Here are some other fun facts on teen pregnancy to warm your heart and get you fired up:

2 out of 3 Number of total teen pregnancies that occur among 18-19 year olds. That's right after they graduate from high school, move out of your house and away from your watchful eye.[12]

1 out of 7: Sexually active girls under the age of 15 who will become pregnant.[13]

27: Percentage of teen pregnancies that end in abortion.[14]

Teen parents are more likely to become dependent on welfare, to live in poverty and drop out of high school.[15]

51: Percentage of teen moms that go on to get their high school diploma or GED, compared to 89% of teen girls who did not have a child.[16]

New Mexico leads the country with 93 out of every one thousand teens becoming pregnant, followed by Nevada, Arizona, Texas and Mississippi.[17]

You may have already covered all this, or you planted a seed once upon a time and now it's appropriate to go into more detail.

Below are some talking points to kick-start this discussion with your daughter and son

1. Male sexual organs and what are they called, as well as various functions.
2. What is an erection and how does it happen?
3. What is the difference between precum, semen and sperm?
4. How long can sperm survive in a woman's uterus after ejaculation? (3 to 5 days)
5. Women's sexual organs and what they are called, as well as their various functions.
6. What happens each month when a woman ovulates and then menstruates?
7. How does a woman get pregnant?
8. When is a woman most likely to get pregnant?*

* When she is ovulating, which is always 14 days before her period begins. But because sperm can stay in the uterus 3-5 days, sex before or after could still result in a pregnancy if there is an ejaculation.

Chapter 7: Physical Impact

When your parents were having sex (don't think about that, it will just weird you out), there were two main Sexually Transmitted Diseases (STD): Syphilis and Gonorrhea. Today, your child can pick from one of about 27. Only they don't get to pick. The STD picks them. In this age of political correctness, you can be sure these little critters are very progressive and have jumped on the equal-opportunity bandwagon with gusto. They do not discriminate according to a person's sexual orientation, gender, age, race, religion, cleanliness, socio-economic status, popularity or sobriety. If they find a warm body, they will seriously consider sending their own Mayflower. Even if that warm body is your son or daughter.

If you want to hunt down the entire list of STDs, be my guest. A good place to start would be the Center for Disease Control's site, www.cdc.gov. For those of you who have to get to carpool soon, here are my "Fab

Four" for you to know and bring up tonight at dinner with your teenagers. Pictures are optional.

1. Chlamydia & Gonorrhea: Chlamydia is currently the most frequently reported bacterial STD, although teens and young adults report the highest rates of infection for Gonorrhea.[18] These two bacterial infections are very similar in their symptoms, though not identical. While antibiotics can clear up both of these, if left untreated in females they can develop into Pelvic Inflammatory Disease (PID). The bacteria causes scar tissue in the fallopian tubes, leading either to infertility or possibly an ectopic pregnancy in the future.[19] Symptoms tend to be mild or non-existent but the serious irreversible damage can still occur internally. Those fortunate enough to show symptoms will have yellow or greenish discharge that may smell like dead fish. So if you notice your child or one of their friends starting to smell like the local fish market (and they don't hang out there regularly), get them to a clinic or doctor. Hope that didn't just ruin your lunch.

2. Genital Herpes: There is currently no cure for Genital Herpes (as opposed to bacteria, which can be cleared up with antibiotics), one of the most common viral infections in the US. This means that regardless of when your child becomes infected, it will be with them for the rest of their life. Take note: one in six Americans has Genital Herpes, or an estimated 45 million people.[20]

If your son or daughter chooses to be sexually active with multiple partners, it is not a question of IF but WHEN they will encounter this virus and whether they will know it. Like many of these STDs, most infected people do not show symptoms but are still contagious. Don't believe me? I have two friends with genital herpes. One broke out at 21 but has no idea who gave it to her. Her boyfriend at the time didn't have it, and she never saw anything on her other partners to give her concern. My second friend was lucky enough to have the guy she was with actually tell her he had the Herp. But he incorrectly informed her that as long as he wasn't having an outbreak, she wasn't at risk. A week after having sex, she broke out with ulcers symptomatic of genital herpes.

3. Human Papilloma Virus: The leading cause of cervical cancer in women, this virus has over forty different strains that can be transmitted sexually. In addition to the genital warts it causes, it has been linked to penile, anal and throat cancers in men. It is the most common sexually transmitted infection, and the more partners someone has, the higher the risk. HPV is also highly contagious through skin-to-skin contact, fluid, and mucus.

Unfortunately, as I write this there is currently no FDA approved test for HPV in men. Unless he breaks out with warts, there is really no way for a woman to know if the man she is dating has any of these strains. If he has had multiple partners, there is a greater risk, since men are more often carriers and don't show symptoms. Unlike the other viruses mentioned here, ninety percent of HPV cases will clear themselves up within a couple of years.[21] The question is, will your child get one of the ninety percent, or the ten percent that don't clear themselves up, leading to further complications?[1]

Gardasil is a vaccine available as a preventative measure. Since I'm not a medical professional, and I'm not about to wade into that political quagmire, I'm very careful to neither recommend nor discourage the HPV vaccine. Whether or not to have the shot is a decision to be made by each parent according to what they see as best for their child.

---

[1] The vaccination for HPV, Gardasil, protects about 80% of the time against the four most serious strains of the virus, the two that are leading causes of cervical cancer and the two that are the leading causes of genital warts. The shot is only effective if given *before* your child encounters HPV and remember, it still leaves them open to another 36 strains.

I encourage you to research the vaccine, to look at the recommendations made by the CDC, then speak with your child's doctor and talk with other parents.

Keep in mind as you are deciding what to do that: a) the HPV vaccine is not necessary for young people if they are not sexually active because, b) it is meant to protect against the four leading strains of sexually transmitted HPV that cause genital warts and cervical cancer. If your son is not sexually active, there is no risk of him contracting the virus and therefore no reason for him to get the shot. If he is sexually active or is going to be in the future, the shot does reduce the risk of contracting four out of the forty strains of HPV that can be transmitted sexually. But it does nothing to protect against other STDs. Make sure that your child knows this. Only you, as the parent, can decide what is best for your child's health. This includes the expectations you want to set, and the message you are sending by choosing whether or not to get the shot.

4. HIV/AIDS: Perhaps the STD we are most familiar with (thank you Bono and the Red Campaign), this one makes this list because it is still a threat to young people, and still deadly.* To date, there is still no cure for the

* www.joinred.com

virus. Expensive medications can prolong the amount of time before HIV develops into full-blown AIDS but it still means a drastically reduced life span. Not to mention a lifestyle now controlled by a rigid regiment of drugs. A condom, when used consistently and correctly, protects eighty-five percent of the time.[22]

This leaves your child with a one in six chance of getting a deadly virus every time they engage in sexual activity with a new partner. If they have another STD, such as Gonorrhea or Genital Herpes, they are two to five times more likely to contract HIV when they encounter it than someone who does not have a preexisting STD.[23] Risky behavior leads to riskier behavior. Don't stay up late at night worrying about this, but also don't dismiss this as, "That problem in Africa."

This list of "Fab Four" are not meant to scare you, but simply make you aware of the very real physical risks your child could encounter, and how it will impact them both now and in the future.

Many teens do not realize that when they engage in sexual activity with someone, they are exposed not only to that partner, but also to every person that partner has ever been with. Messing around with one or two people may not seem to pose much risk, until you consider how many partners that person has had, and how many partners their partners have had. The numbers can add up pretty quickly.

Some of you are already getting distracted counting up your own partners. Stop it! Focus.

I'd like to tell you a little story about Sally. I illustrated this myself, so prepare to be amazed.

This is Sally.

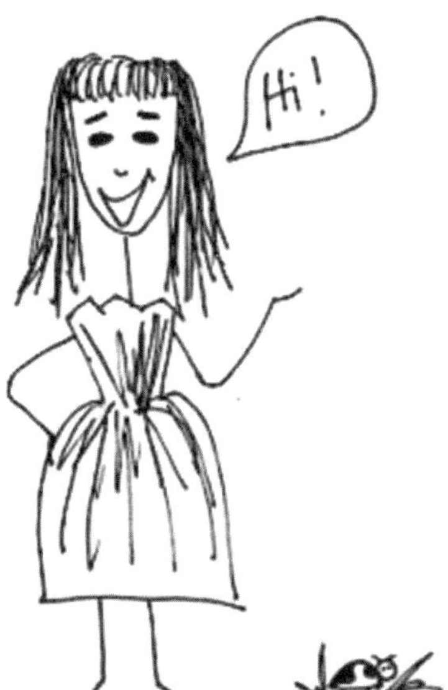

Freshman year of High School...

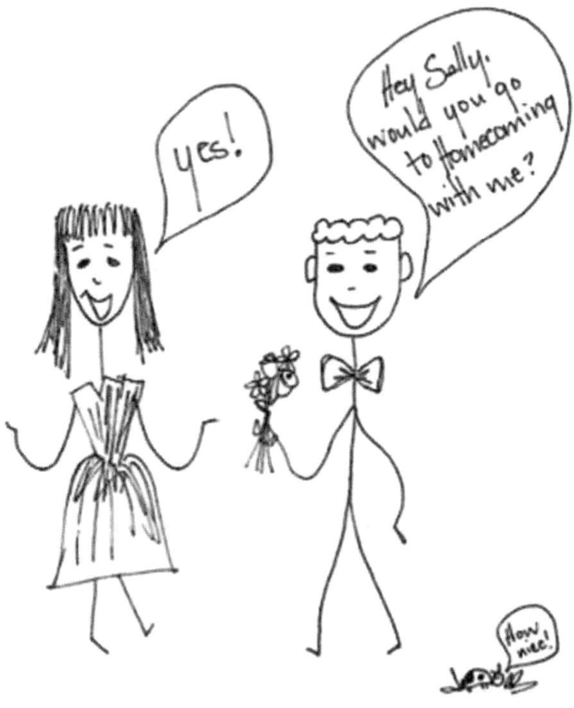
yes!
Hey Sally, would you go to Homecoming with me?
How nice!

Result: Skin-on-skin contact
(clothes off but no sex)

Exposure Count total: 1

Sophomore year, Sally gets a boyfriend...

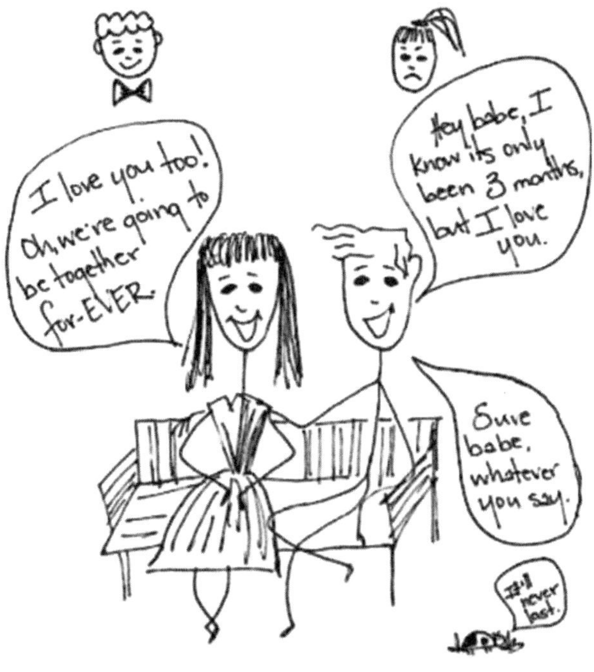
I love you too! Oh, we're going to be together for-EVER.
Hey babe, I know its only been 3 months, but I love you.
Sure babe, whatever you say.
It'll never last.

Result: Sexual intercourse
(They're in love!)

Exposure Count total: 3

End of junior year, Sally gets dumped...

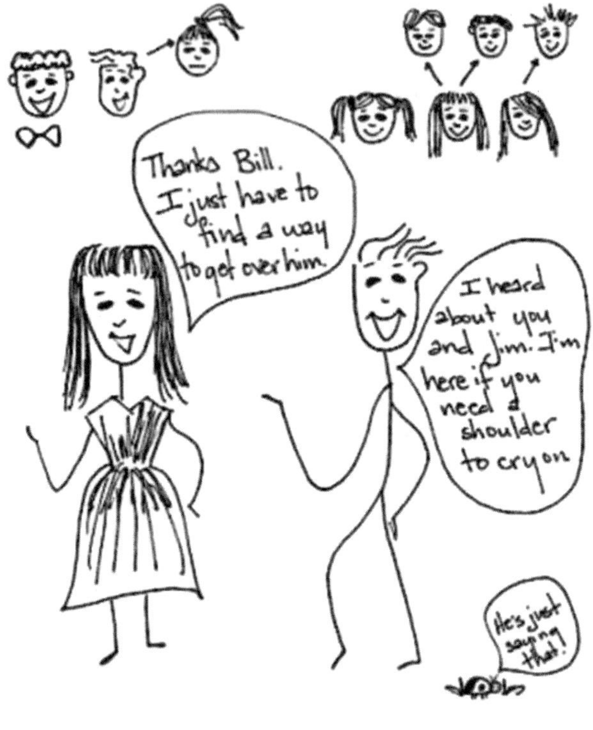
Thanks Bill. I just have to find a way to get over him.
I heard about you and Jim. I'm here if you need a shoulder to cry on
He's just saying that!

Result: Sexual Intercourse
(Revenge! Or is it Rebound?)

Exposure Count total: 10

Senior Year, Sally goes to a party…

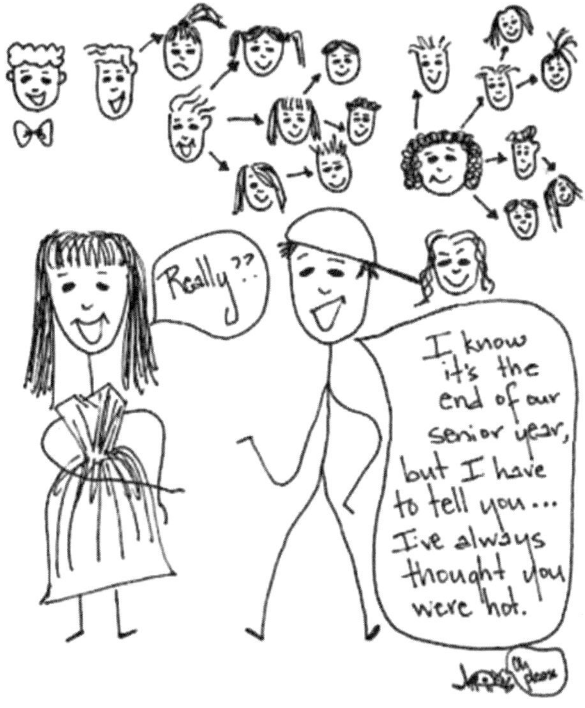
Really??
I know it's the end of our senior year, but I have to tell you… I've always thought you were hot.

Result: Oral Sex
(It's safer than 'real' sex, right?)

Exposure Count total: 20

Finally, Sally goes off to college...

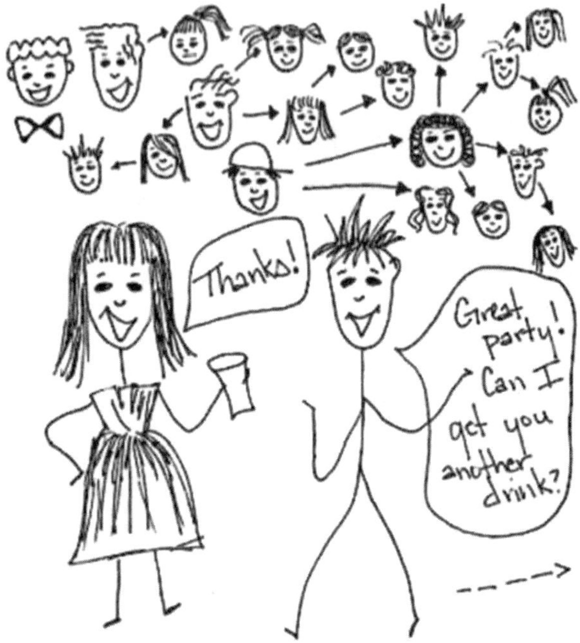

Result: Genital skin to skin contact, possibly oral sex?

(The details are a bit hazy)

Exposure Count Total: 39

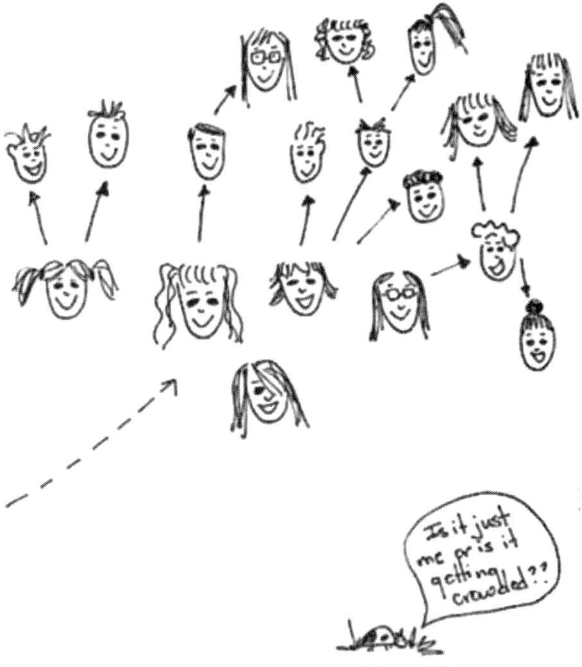

Clearly I should stick to writing over drawing, but wasn't that a nice little story? Sally only had a handful of partners and they all looked clean to her, so clearly, she wasn't at much risk for contracting an STD. I have no doubt she'll find a wonderful man, get married someday, and live happily ever after.

But it wasn't just those 5. There are thirty-four other individuals she was also exposed to, thirty-four individuals that she never had the opportunity to ask about their sexual history and habits, about their other partners, and whether or not they got tested regularly. This assumes Sally was smart enough to ask her own five partners about their history and to demand STD testing.

Unfortunately, this is not the case for most teens and even young adults who merely depend on the "Look Test" to gauge their risk, (looks fine, let's go!).

This story may not be Pulitzer Prize worthy, but it's a clever way to help your child understand that it is not one for one when it comes to their risk for an STD. For every person they are physically with, either through genital skin-to-skin contact, oral, anal, or vaginal sex, they are also exposed to that person's previous partners.

Call them over, right now, and say, "Hey, look at this weird little story in this book I'm reading. Did you know this? It's kind of crazy!" You can literally say this word for word.

What this story fails to measure is the emotional risk from each new partner, the attachments formed and the memories. You don't forget that first person you had sex with, even if they're 8 people back. You don't erase every regrettable sexual encounter, and you cannot prevent your heart and brain from bonding. More on that in a moment.

Chapter 8: Latex Parachutes and Other Safety Measures

Ok, so there's risk. BUT we have an answer for that, right? Condoms and birth control! Condoms definitely reduce a person's risk for contracting an STD (make sure your teen knows that birth control offers NO protection against STDs) and should be used if someone is sexually active outside of a committed relationship, such as marriage. But as you learned in your intro quiz, they only offer about fifty percent protection when used consistently and correctly.[24] Even less for HPV because it is so contagious through skin-to-skin contact. It reduces risk, which is good, but it doesn't remove risk, which is what many teens mistakenly believe. Why not, you may ask? Simple.

Latex boxer briefs haven't been invented yet.

Condoms don't really cover all that much (no offense, gentlemen). Yes, they cover the penis or can line the vagina, but what about the other skin surrounding those areas? Those are still exposed and vulnerable to infection. If skin-to-skin contact by itself can put someone at risk for an STD, then this still holds true when there's that and more coming by being in "closer" contact.

Birth control pills, patches and rings, IUDS, and the Depo Provera shot, can prevent against pregnancy 95-99% of the time-a woman's doctor can recommend what is best for her lifestyle, body, and general health.[25] Condoms, if used consistently and correctly, come in at about 85%.[26] Any and all of these are available options for reducing the risk of pregnancy and STDs.

But none of these options offers a guaranteed one hundred percent rate of protection. Even if we could create a condom that was 97% fool-proof, covering all of your teens nether regions, we would still be leaving our kids vulnerable.

How so, you ask?

There's no condom for your heart.

Neither is there a pill to diminish attachment, a patch or a shot to turn your heart off in the moment. There's no way to prevent you from bonding with someone outside of a healthy, committed relationship like marriage.

This is why simply educating about condoms, birth control, teen pregnancy and STDs leaves your kids cheated, with only half of the story. An important half, but nevertheless, half. Too many of our teens are finding out far too late that a broken heart and unwanted memories can be just as serious as an STD.

67 Percent of teens wish they had waited longer before having sex.[27]

No matter how many times they're told that as long as they use a condom they'll be safe, that it's not that big of a deal, or that this is a healthy and natural part of growing up...they are still finding out that it IS a big deal, that it DOES matter and that there are some things a condom cannot protect against.

Before you write me off as a sentimental looney, allow me to pull back the curtain on what is behind the great and powerful emotions of sex. It will blow your mind.

Next sextion please. I mean, section.

Chapter 9: Going Emo* on Your Kids

There are two chemicals that your brain releases to create bonding between you and other people, including between your sexual partner(s) and you. Ladies, you only release Oxcytocin and gentlemen, you release both Oxcytocin and Vasopressin. Gents, you get this second bonding chemical because unlike sea horses, you don't get nine months of pregnancy. So you miss out on that oh so special experience with your child. Referred to as the "Monogamy Molecule," this chemical also serves to strengthen the bond between you and your spouse. Bonus.

Triggers for these chemical releases are as follows (1 & 2 are obviously limited to one gender. I'll let you take a guess which one):

1. Onset of labor during a pregnancy

---

* Emotional: to be in touch with one's emotions; punk-angst attitude that some teens adopt for way too long.

2. Breastfeeding
3. Meaningful or intimate touch
4. Sexual intercourse

Meaningful or intimate touch can obviously look very different depending on the relationship. Between your kids and you, it might be playing around, hugging, curling up together to watch a movie or that kiss you smack on their cheek as they're running out the door. With your spouse, meaningful and intimate touch is going to include a lot more, such as foreplay and sexual activity. In the context of your child's sexual relationships, it's....all of those same things. So your kid may not go all the way, but if they're passionately kissing, getting naked, giving or receiving oral...you get the idea. Through all of it, they're releasing varying degrees of these chemicals, causing your child to trust that other person, want more of them, and desire to be around them more.

You'll notice 'Sexual Intercourse' got its own number on the list. That's because sex literally takes things to a whole other level. If your son or daughter chooses to "go all the way," their brain releases five times the amount of Oxcytocin that it normally would. Five times!

Their brain is literally flooded with these chemicals that burn little neurological pathways into their brain to connect them with that person.

I told you it was amazing! And I don't even like science. Now, all of this bonding is great when you're married, but not so great when you're 16 years old.* A person's brain does not know how to distinguish between prom night (a one night stand) and someone's wedding night. It doesn't know when this isn't a person to bond with or when this is part of a life-long committed relationship. It just knows the triggers, and boom! The floodgates open.

Let's think back to the story about Sally. Does it matter all that much for your son or daughter's brain/heart as long as their body count of connecting partners stays somewhere in the single digits? New science on the brain is showing the painful result that casual sexual encounters are having on today's teens. Their brain is still forming (which explains why they sometimes act like they're missing half of it) and will continue to do so until they're in their twenties. If they build a habit of short, physically intense relationships, they can actually mold and train their brain to *only* engage in short,

* If you're married and reading this, please go have sex with your spouse tonight. Your relationship will be the better for it.

physically intense relationships. When it comes time for them to form a long-term commitment, such as marriage, their brain literally does not know how to switch gears. It has been damaged by the cycle of connection and break-up.[28]

This applies to girls *and* guys. It's not just the ladies forming this emotional bond and the sons who get off without a second thought. They are just as affected, especially when it comes to the habits and pathways formed in their brain. While not irreversible, the habits and pathways formed in their brain from repeated sexual encounters can be difficult to unlearn. It will take a concerted effort on their part to behave differently in their future relationships than in their past, but only if they understand why they are inclined to act a certain way.

Not only does your child risk damaging their ability to create a strong, long lasting bond in the future, but they can experience the following emotional fall-outs today from being sexually active.

- Broken Heart: The same place in the brain that feels physical pain can also feel pain from a broken relationship and rejection. So heartbreak does hurt.[29]

- Regret: Of sexually active teens, six out of ten say they wish they had waited longer. When you break it down by gender, it comes out at roughly the same: 65% of girls and 57% of boys.[30]

- A negative effect on their reputation: this can lead to bullying, taunting and name calling at school.

- Depression: Teens who have had sex are three times more likely to be depressed than friends who are virgins[31]

- Suicidal Thoughts: Sexually active girls are three times more likely to have attempted suicide than their virgin friends, while sexually active guys are *seven times* more likely.[32]

Side note: If you notice your child has suddenly become very withdrawn, moody, or emotional, it could have something to do with having been in a relationship and/or being physically intimate with someone and then that relationship ending. You need to talk to them in a way that makes them feel safe, and lets them know you're there to listen, whatever the conversation may be.

Relationships are tough stuff. But they are also the golden threads that bring beauty to the tapestry of our lives (poetic, right?). This need to talk to your kids about sex and relationships is because you're trying to set them up to succeed, to minimize or even avoid some of these consequences, and to help equip them to make choices that will allow them to live their life to the fullest.

You know what all this means? It means that we are each wired to bond with one person, to literally become addicted. Crazy, I know. But beautiful too. And if you're tearing at your hair right now to get to those ill-fated neurological pathways you formed during your knucklehead years, have no fear. The brain is an amazing organ and can actually reform and repair itself. It can be an arduous and prolonged process, but it is possible. But how much better for your son or daughter to be spared the pain, and simply enjoy bonding with abandon to that one person they can safely trust with their heart forever?

Chapter 10: I'm a Digital Girl, Living In a Digital World

The world has changed quite a bit since you were 16 years old, a fact your teen or pre-teen rarely lets you forget. We're going faster, filling our schedules more tightly, and multitasking every moment we're not sleeping. We have music, phones, computers, and TVs blazing 24/7 as we travel through life. With the touch of a button, you have access to more information than the National Archives could ever contain. Paper has been replaced by digital, which is why some of you are reading this on tablets, smart phones and computers. Others of you have no idea what I just said. Don't worry, you'll catch up.

TV

By the time your baby graduates from high school, they will have spent an average of 15,000 hours in front of the Tube. Need some perspective on how much time that is? That institution of learning that you send them to

Monday through Friday (with some of you already paying the equivalent of college tuition rates) will consume 11,000 hours of their life by the time they put on one of those terrible polyester robes and march out to Pomp and Circumstance. At the small cost of your monthly cable bill over those same 13+ years, you get the 11,000 hours of screen time PLUS a bonus four thousand hours. If you suddenly have a strong urge to run into the other room, turn the TV off and kick your kids outside, I don't blame you. But before you do, let's consider, for a moment, exactly what they're being taught in those 625 accumulated days of staring into that glowing box.

In the course of just one year, your teen will be exposed to an average of 14,000 instances of sexual material on TV. If you limit them to only the Food Network or the Disney Channel you're looking at probably a whopping 23 instances.

As they get older you may be less inclined to check in on what your teens are watching. Don't. First of all, if you have younger kids, it is inevitable they will, at some point, sit down with your older child to watch the same show. Who doesn't want to be just like their big brother or sister? Secondly, the messages being glammed up and pumped out in 95% of shows don't exactly provide a balanced and well-educated look at sexuality.[4] Fairly one-sided in their approach, they do a great job of casting those who choose not to have sex as the ugly losers (which therefore implies their lack of sex), while it is the sexually active who are beautiful, popular and oh-so-enlightened. After all, it's when you're like, totally smart, that you like, know that as long as you use a condom there are *no* risks to sex except falling madly in love and making your relationship much stronger!

What the creators and the distributors of these shows won't tell you about is a study released in 2008 showing that teens who watch television shows with high levels of sexual content are twice as likely to become pregnant over the next three years than those who watched fewer such programs.[33]

With all of this sexually saturated programming, it might surprise you to hear that 61% of kids state they want to be virgins when they get married, and 52% will graduate high school never having had sexual intercourse. The problem is you won't hear many of them proudly voicing this.[34] I have teens tell me weekly that they don't want to have sex yet because they have other things they're focusing on, that they want to wait until they're in a committed relationship, or even married. And by committed, they don't mean 6 months during sophomore year. But try to get them to take an outspoken stand on this and for the most part you'll only hear radio silence. They don't want to look like losers by the standards of a social script spoken every day on dozens of their favorite TV shows.

Now you may go shut the TV off.

In addition to the hours they will spend in front of the TV, there is the time they spend online on social networking sites, emailing, using Hulu to catch up on the shows they forgot to TiVo, hours frittered away on YouTube (if you've seen one laughing baby, you've seen them all, yet we keep watching, and watching and watching). Experts at digital multitasking, the average 8-18 year old daily crams about 10 hours and 45 minutes worth of media content into 7 1/2 hours.[35] That's more time than they spend at school!

Keeping all those stats in mind, I have to ask: Do you care as much about what your children are learning from all those hours with the media as you do about their formal education? (If you're currently not involved in their school life, that doesn't mean you keep doing nothing. Step it up!). When was the last time you sat down with them while they were watching a show? And have you noticed how they are using media to promote themselves, to craft a message to the world about who they are? That means on their Facebook page, through their tweets, in chat rooms and if they have a phone, via texting. Lots and lots of texting...

CELL PHONES & SOCIAL MEDIA

If your child has a phone or a device (such as an itouch or iPad) that allows them to send and receive text messages then you need to keep reading. The rest of you can take a five minute break to go grab a drink. Of....water.

75 Percent of 12-17 year-olds that now own cell phones.

Half of teens send **50+ texts a day.**

1 in 3 teens send more than one-hundred texts/day, or three thousand texts/month.

3000+ texts/month: Typical amount sent by a 14-17 year old girl. [36]

There's quite a bit of angst about the number of teens sexting. In case you're in the dark about that particular new term, 'sexting' is a way of referring to the sexually explicit texts sent and received by teenagers. It can range from something written, to pictures depicting partial or full nudity.

A study in 2009 put the number of teens that have sent nude or seminude photos as high as twenty percent. Some of you may have heard that and panicked, certain that the world was going to hell in a hand basket. Have I got good news for you! A study came out in Fall 2011 that restricted the definition of what was nude or semi-nude to only that which was sexually explicit (i.e. showed naked breasts, genitals or bottoms). In doing so they found that....are you ready for it... one percent of kids between 10-17 years of age have sent those types of photos. One percent. When the definition was expanded for beach style fashion, it grew to 2.5%.

7.1 Percent of teens have received nude or semi-nude images of others.

5.9 Percent of teens have received sexually explicit images (the narrower definition).[37]

Now don't you feel better? At least until you think about your child being that one percent. Then it might as well be 90%. Or until you remember that those numbers only deal with sexually explicit *images*.

What about those written texts and emails that would make Grandma blush?

48 Percent of teens say they have received sexually suggestive messages.[38]

For kids who have grown up in a culture where leaked sex tapes lead to overnight fame and fortune, it's hard for them to see why the above statistics are disconcerting. They fail to connect that the ease with which they sent that picture to the cute boy in their geometry class also means that same image could go viral to thousands, in mere minutes. Hardly a second thought is given to what this could mean for their reputation, or how it could come back to haunt them years down the road. This might be the very thing they've needed to become the next Paris Hilton or Kim Kardashian!

That thought alone is going to give some of you nightmares tonight.

You know that whatever gets posted online is there forever. Or if you didn't, you do now. Does your son know that? I mean, *really* know that? Does your daughter fully grasp what sort of a reputation she creates when she posts certain pictures or writes certain things in texts or on people's wall? One hundred and forty characters may not seem like much, but it can do some serious damage these days. A picture is worth a thousand words, not all of them good ones.

Facebook. YouTube. Twitter. Instagram. Foursquare. Tumbler. Vimeo. These have changed the way we "do" relationships, how we interact with the world around us, and the identity we build for ourselves. Even as you're teaching your son or daughter how to have real flesh and blood relationships with face-to-face human interaction, you need to be wise to the fact that they are digitally creating an image for themselves.

Just because you're not the most media savvy parent out there doesn't mean you cannot or should not be discussing this with your child. You didn't think you could talk about sex, and you're still reading! Anything is possible at this point. You may not completely understand how Twitter works or what it means to retweet, hashtag or poke, but you do understand that actions have consequences – never more so than in this age of 24/7 news.

Some questions to consider:

Facebook/Twitter/Social Networking Sites

If your child has a page on any of these sites, have you taken a look at it lately?

If they are under the age of fifteen, do you know the password, and how to change their privacy settings?

If they are over the age of fifteen, have you discussed and agreed on appropriate privacy settings?

What is your and your child's policy on who to connect with online, and what requests are acceptable?

Have you discussed what pictures are appropriate or what is acceptable to write on a person's wall, to tweet, or who to follow?

Anything that is written is easily forwarded, shared and seen by others so your son or daughter needs to be conscious of what they are saying and what image they are creating.

Texting

What should they do if they receive an inappropriate text?

If your child is an avid texter, do they help pay for that?

Do you have a limit on how much texting is allowed, perhaps because of your cell phone plan?

What is appropriate to text and what is not? What might be some of the dangers of texting certain messages or images?

Have you discussed the ease with which someone could forward a message or picture and how that could affect them?

Do some exploratory work first to become familiar with some of these social media components, so you have a base knowledge when speaking to your child. Set up your own profiles, "friend" your kid and start following them – digitally that is. You still don't get to stalk them throughout their day. If you really want some laughs, ask them to help you set all this up. It'll be a riot. At least for them. Until they realize the monster they've released in you, as you become a social networking fiend.

You'll also be able to friend, follow, and tweet me, meaning I'm just a few clicks away from your beck and call. As long as it's between the hours of 9-5 PST, Monday through Friday.

Chapter 11: Pornography - Yes, You Have to Talk About It. No, It's Not Optional.

Pornography is a multi-billion dollar industry that is incredibly easy for people to access. It used to be that you would have to get in your car and drive to an adult bookstore or a gas station to pick up your porn of choice. Or hope you had a very discreet mail delivery person who could keep your secret. There was always the risk that people who knew you might see you. It cost you something in time, money and potentially, in reputation. You had to put some effort into getting that pornography!

These days, it's as easy as the click of a button from the comfort of your home. It's often free, and whatever you're looking for, you'll find it. You can even stumble upon it while innocently searching something else. All of a sudden, wham! There it is, in your face, uninvited. To be honest, just watch a little mainstream TV or check out some billboards and you're sure to get a sampling of flesh.

The numbers are staggering in terms of how much money is made each year by the porn industry, how many people are looking at it, the number of websites, and the avid teen usage. Clearly we have a problem. Consider these numbers a conservative estimate. With how rapidly the pornography industry is growing, it is difficult to get an exact estimate.

Every second: $3,075.64 is being spent on pornography.

Every 39 minutes: a new pornographic video is being created in the United States.

89 Percent of sexual solicitations of youth are made in chat rooms.

90 Percent of 8-19 year olds have viewed pornography.[39]

Shocked? Good. Please feel free to refer back to these numbers whenever your resolve begins to waver on talking to your child about porn. They'll give you the nerves of steel you need.

But wait, is it a problem? You've no doubt heard the arguments that everyone needs a little visual stimulation now and then, that pornography can help jump start a stalled relationship or help a couple get creative in the bedroom. It's a way for us (adults and teens alike) to compartmentalize sex into our busy lives, to meet our 'need' for sexual release without risk of an STD, pregnancy, or awkward encounter the next morning. To say it's addicting or harmful to an individual or a couple is just being extreme. This is art, self-expression, glorification of the human body!

For those of you that have only daughters, don't you dare think you can skip this section or this discussion. The number of girls viewing and becoming addicted to pornography is growing. Not to mention that your daughters should be taught how much women are objectified, degraded and even harmed during this trash 'art,' and that they do not need to put up with or participate in this within their own relationships. Yes, I have an opinion on this. If you disagree, that's fine. We can still be friends.

With an estimated thirty percent of women and seventy percent of men looking at porn, (and those are often conservative estimates) this would mean that some perfectly healthy, highly functioning individuals we encounter every day are looking at it.[40] Including some of you reading these words. *Uncomfortable pause.* Is it just me or did it get a little, um, tense, around here? I'll tread carefully. In order for you to be able to help your child live a healthy, successful life when it comes to sex and relationships, YOU are going to have to do the same, both publicly and privately. Pornography can become highly addictive. It's not easily contained in the private corner of your life; it sends ripples and repercussions into other areas.

I am not saying everyone who views pornography is addicted. Although if you're getting all huffy and upset with me right now, you might want to think about what that means. A person who looks at pornography regularly but claims not to be addicted should try to go one week without looking. One. I give this same challenge to the teens with whom I speak.

For you to understand why pornography can have such a powerful hold on people, we need to peel back the skull to get a look at what is going on inside the brain, and why this warrants a discussion with your child.

The Control Center of our bodies, each of our brains, has a Reward System that helps us remember the things that we like, whether they be food, people, sounds, visual stimulation or experiences, as well as how we got to those stimulators. The main chemical in this system is Dopamine. This little chemical is released in each of us every day in small amounts, creating our threshold, or ground floor starting level. When something new or exciting enters our day, we get a shot of Dopamine to the brain that helps us remember exactly how we got to that something new – to remember what it was that gave us such enjoyment. This rush creates a feeling of ecstasy and exhilaration: it's totally dope. Although don't say it that way to your kids, unless you want to lose some serious coolness points.

Our brain is crazy smart so it also remembers what was going on around us when it got that shot of dopamine: smells, sounds, tastes, places. Being around any of these same things can trigger Dopamine, giving us a craving for more. A person who looks at pornography & masturbates might be determined to leave that in the past and then almost without notice, find themselves right back at it. They're not even quite sure how they got there! Something triggered that chemical release and reminded them (even if they were not aware) that the last time they felt that high, that rush, they were looking at porn/masturbating. So they instinctively go back to it in order to fill the craving.

In addition to the rush, dopamine also slows down our decision making skills, making it difficult to judge what the best choice is in that moment. Which explains the risks your teen is perpetually inclined to take! It is also why they may find it difficult to resist when the dopamine starts pumpin', even though they know they tend to feel guilty, empty, and even shameful when the experience is over. Their brain is only thinking about how good they feel in the moment, not how they're going to feel afterwards.

Remember the two other chemicals I mentioned earlier? The ones that are intended for bonding during sexual arousal? Yeah, they join the party too. Except the bonding and sense of intimacy is with a leggy... picture, or the person on their screen. Both of which have been airbrushed, edited, pumped and pinned up to create an alternate reality: a reality where the individual does not have feelings, problems, demands or issues. A reality where the relationship is purely sexual and one-sided. Whether you are currently married, or have been in the past, you know that is the furthest thing from reality! Every pizza delivery girl does NOT want to have sex. Neither is every girl walking around dying for a guy to ask her to have some sort of crazy, kinky sex. Pornography paints false expectations about relationships, sex, and dealing with other people, ultimately undermining a person's ability to have a healthy relationship and eventually, a healthy marriage.

All this chemical bonding and memory burning that occurs means quitting cold turkey is much harder than "Just say No." The brain has learned to respond to certain triggers, to become addicted to particular behaviors. Like most addictions, the brain builds up a tolerance to the dopamine, requiring a greater stimulant to feel the same rush. The soft core porn someone started with will no longer provide the same feeling of euphoria and they'll find themselves slowly escalating and expanding to more and more explicit images, increasing how often they seek out those images. With the average age of exposure for guys somewhere around 11 years old, this is a topic that should be at the top of your priority list.*

How you approach the subject of pornography is ultimately up to you. But it needs to be discussed.

---

* I've read some reports that drop that age to eight years old. I want to be surprised but sadly, I just can't. Hello world that we're living in.

Here are some aspects to cover:

- Talk about how pornography exploits women.
- Explain how it portrays a false reality about sex and relationships.
- Engage them in dialogue about how it could effect their relationships, such as having to explain to their future husband or wife that this is something to which they are addicted.
- Educate them on how cool their brain is...and what pornography does to it.
- Be proactive in helping your children avoid the temptation by putting the computer in a public place in the house.
- Install software that blocks certain sites and sets parameters on the amount of time someone can spend online and what they can do.

It's a tough pill to swallow, but the reality is that while many of our children may look like the perfect models of purity on the outside, by avoiding all outward display of sexual activity or risk, they're still addicted to pornography. If ninety percent of 8-19 year olds have viewed pornography, then it's very likely your child is one of them. Whether or not they're still viewing and hiding it from you is another question.

Your teenager needs to be reminded regularly, in words and actions, that your love is not based on their meeting certain standards or projecting a certain image. You will love them no matter what they do, and are there to help them if they are or ever do find themselves struggling. If your son or daughter does come to you and admit they need help, there are plenty of resources out there, some of which I've mentioned under the **Resources** section in the back of the book. A good place to start is to help them identify what it is that triggers that desire to look at porn and/or masturbate – such as being home by themselves, bored, getting in a fight with you, talking to a particular friend, etc. Together you can begin retraining the brain and actively watching for triggers.

This isn't a problem that is exclusive to teens. Adults, both male and female, struggle with addictions to pornography at alarming rates. While the focus of this book is how to talk to your kids about sex, it may be that some of *you* need to access those resources and begin to address your own addiction to pornography.

As I'll cover later in the book, your example is paramount in making these conversations successful. It's never too late to start practicing sexual integrity and bring healing into potentially damaged relationships.

Chapter 12: Relationships, like Death and Taxes, are Inevitable

At some point your teen is going to get asked out on a date. Or do the asking.

As much as you may like to prevent that from happening until they're 23, accept the fact that they are going to go on at least one date with at least one person in the near future. Eventually, they'll go on a lot of dates with one person who they likely will choose to marry. Which is a good thing. So unless you're planning on arranging their marriage (which I don't foresee going over well), this is a milestone in their life that you will have to face. Together.

The good news:

Talking about relationships is fun! Of all the things you 'get' to discuss with your son or daughter relating to sex, talking about relationships will likely be the least awkward and the most of fun of all.

Picture it: This a chance for you to share a few horror stories of your own (we *all* have at least one terrible first date story), to laugh over those gender differences that are both infuriating and endearing (why do girls go to the bathroom in groups? Or like to talk about shopping *so* much?), and give your child the tools needed to have a good time, while staying safe.

Maybe this only sounds fun to me, not you. But when it comes to the questions teens have, you might be surprised (and relieved) how many of them have to do with love, emotions, boys, girls, dating, asking someone out, how to know if she likes me, why he doesn't call me the next day; the typical stuff of relationships that everyone deals with until they're married or dead I guess.

We know that girls are all about relationships. Isn't that why we find that many of them will give in to sex sooner than they would have liked? They want to keep the relationship, or hope to finally make it official. But that is only half of the story. In a study of young men between 15-18 years old, 71% said that they would rather have a girlfriend and no sex rather than sex and no relationships.[41] So relationships matter to our young men as well. More so than sex. I know, shocking. Pick your jaw up off the floor and let's keep moving.

It's obvious then, what you need to do.

....

No...?

If our teens are telling us that given the choice, they would prefer a committed relationship over sex, than you need to be talking about that as much as you are talking about sex. Or not having sex. Or at least waiting. You get the point. If your child is aiming to postpone sexual activity until a committed relationship such as marriage, and they actually value relationships, they need to first understand how to build said relationship. It does not happen over-night. And with all due respect to teens, it does not come naturally to them. Let's be honest, does it come naturally to many of us? We all have broken relationships in our past. And for better or worse, they make us who we are. Your teen will probably have a relationship disaster or two by the time they marry. You can minimize the depth and duration, and give them a head start, by teaching the following five aspects of relationships.

1. Dating Basics

Chivalry is not dead. At least not as long as I have a say in it. But I won't get very far if I'm the only one to champion it. You need to be teaching your son or daughter the basics: basics of how a guy should treat a girl when he takes her out, of how a girl should handle herself on a date. Basics of respect. Or dating. The same thing, really. Don't just talk about this one, live it. My dad opened doors for me and my mom and walked on the outside of the street when we'd go out. I'm a bit ashamed to admit that I went through a phase of yelling at boys for opening the door for me. I've done lots of apologizing since. How was I supposed to know at 13 that it was a sign of respect, not a statement on female inferiority??

Somewhere I did, however, learn to never order a more expensive item than the guy taking me out ordered. And while I'd offer to help pay for dinner, I expected that if this was a date then he should pay. No going Dutch. Unless I had done the asking of course. Which I didn't. At least not the first date.

Does your son know not to ask a girl out through Facebook? Or text? Does your daughter expect a guy to come to the door to pick her up, not just honk the horn? What about appropriate conversation topics and how to actually have a conversation i.e. Ask questions about the other person and be interested in them, not yourself.

Think I'm old fashioned? Or that these basics don't need to be taught? Ask your daughter what she would want in a date. Not the bare minimum she thinks she can expect, but what she would actually want. Ask your son if he knows these basics. Go ahead, ask.

It seems a bit revolutionary I realize, because the art of dating has been so forgotten and discarded. But if we want to train the next generation to build healthy relationships that will actually go somewhere, we need to bring it back. Vintage is in style these days anyway.

2. Keep the end in mind: Marriage

I realize marriage is probably the last thing on your mind for your child. And certainly the last thing on theirs. Good! Child brides = not cool. I got married at 25 years old and personally, I think that was a lovely age. I've done quite a bit of growing up since then, but I have a sneaking suspicion that marriage will do that to you, no matter what age you are.

My marriage, however, was a decade in the making. Not because I dragged my feet that long or even knew my husband for that many years (although it probably felt like a decade to him because of the work I put him through), but because in my teens I started to think about what kind of a man I would want to marry. Not date, but marry. You'll date a lot of people, but there's only one (hopefully) that you'd be willing to marry.

And not just anyone, but a particular one. The cream of the crop. The one who brings out the best in you and wants to be around for the hard work of improving the worst in each other. Someone you want to spend the rest of your life getting to know, and whose life you want to be around to witness.

That's who we all want to marry. And that's the type of person I would hope you want for your son or daughter. But it won't come from them waking up one day in their twenties and finally starting to look for him or her. They have to have been intentional in their dating, and to have dated with the end in mind. That does not mean a ring on the first coffee date. That's just creepy. And desperate. It means they know who they're looking for because they've thought it through. They are dating to get to know that person and find out whether they are someone worth spending more and more time with, or if it was simply a good date and then a good-bye.

Start asking your child if they've thought about the kind of qualities they would want in someone they would be willing to marry. Begin to discuss what makes someone "marriage material." At seventeen, they're not going to find it. But they may begin to see glimpses. By the time they are in college and especially after, they need to be able to discern whether or not someone is growing in the right direction; if their habits, characteristics and personality are what they are looking for, or if they are trouble waiting to happen.

Some people like to make a list. Fine. If your kid is the list type they can do that, but a word of caution: there is such a thing as expecting too much from a flawed human being, of being unrealistic and putting yourself in a box by sticking rigidly to that list. Don't let your son or daughter get so focused on their "List" that they're unable to let go of what they want for what they need.

As your child begins to think about, and talk about, what qualities they would look for, it should break down into two categories – preferences and core values.

Preferences

This is the wish list of a relationship, everything and the kitchen sink that you want in someone. An ability to cook, musically talented, into the outdoors, tattoo free (ok, maybe that's more yours than theirs), good with kids, likes board games. Whatever. But they're not deal breakers. Your child could meet someone who is actually a terrible cook. But they have a heart of gold. This list (whether written down or not) may change as your child grows and changes, learning what is actually a good fit for them. Great! Each relationship, friend or romantic, is a chance to re-evaluate and re-adjust as they encounter different personalities and people. Open minded is good. Compromising is not.

Core Values

This is a much, much smaller list of qualities or attributes, all of which are deal breakers. If at any point your son or daughter realizes that the person they are dating does not possess one of these, the relationship is off. Harsh? Not at all. We're going for the best here, people. Not sub-par. If your son or daughter really wants to have kids, and the person they are with thinks children are the worst, it's probably not the right fit. Or, if it's important that their spouse be drug-free, then a crack addict isn't the way to go. You get the point. It doesn't mean that the other girl or guy isn't great, just not great for your child.

I always wanted to marry Prince Eric from *The Little Mermaid.* You know the type: tall, dark, handsome, a

Prince. And those were even the guys I tried to date. Except for the prince part – that's a bit hard to find this side of the Atlantic. While they looked good on paper, there was always something lacking. Who did I end up marrying? A 5'9" red head that wears cowboy boots and makes movies. And is the most amazing man I know. Not to mention ridiculously attractive.

If I had made my preferences my core values, I would have missed out on the greatest gift of my life. Make sure that your children know the difference.

3. Red Flags

You don't marry someone to change them. You know that by now. But your son or daughter may not fully grasp that. So when they're dating, they may overlook or dismiss what should be red flags because they think they can either change the person or it's no big deal.

Areas that might raise a red flag:

- How they treat their parents, particularly how a guy treats his mother.
- How someone speaks about ex girlfriends or boyfriends.
- Who they are one on one and who they are in group settings. Are they consistent?

- How that person deals with anger, stress, disappointment.
- How they handle conflict.
- Very different values that could potentially lead to major conflict (faith, family, finances, etc).
- Spending habit, (i.e. they spend everything they make and don't understand the value of money or how to be financially responsible).

Regular conversations with your child will help you discern what is going on in the relationship and allow them time to reflect, as well, on whether or not there is anything that should give them pause. A red flag doesn't mean the relationship is over. It means slow down, take note, discuss and explore a bit further to see whether it's a misunderstanding, a bad day, or the tip of the iceberg to a much bigger problem.

4. The Bad and the Ugly

As much fun as relationships can be, they can also get quite ugly. It is estimated that one in three adolescents in the United States has been a victim of physical, sexual, emotional or verbal abuse from a dating partner. One in ten high school students has been purposefully hit, slapped or physically hurt by their boyfriend or girlfriend.[42] Relationships can turn manipulative, abusive (verbally, physically and sexually) and do serious damage. While some red flags are cause to slow down and reevaluate, others are instant deal breakers.

Does your daughter know she should never put up with being hit or verbally abused? Does your son know that a girl who is extremely jealous, who tries to cut off his other relationships and who gets angry when they're apart is in no way representative of a healthy relationship? Does your child know what to do if they are in a relationship and begin to feel unsafe or uncomfortable? Do they understand that a good relationship has balance, and an unhealthy one is manipulative, controlling, and suffocating? That it's best for them to go into a relationship eyes wide open to what a failing relationship looks like?

It's harder to speak to them when they're in the middle of a bad relationship because they're a bit blinded by emotions. By then, you're the enemy. So be proactive and regularly encourage what your child should be expecting, what is healthy, and how they should be treated. Teach them that they always have a choice, and no degree of abuse is worth putting up with for the sake of being in a relationship.

Begin to empower them with this information now, and when you finally let them date at the age of twenty-five, they'll be ready.

5. Breaking-up. And staying broken up.

Every relationship fails until one does not. That's the brutal truth. Which means that if your son or daughter dates a lot, they will also have to break up a lot. Or at least turn down some dates. But it can be hard to do so, whether for fear of hurting that other person or fear of being alone. Many people would rather stay in a sub-par relationship than break it off completely and risk having to be, (gasp), single!

We all can remember that one couple in high school who was constantly on again, off again. One moment it was sheer glory, the next absolute agony. And I don't just mean for all of us who had to sit next to them in class. I don't know about you, but those couples from my high school didn't get married. They're not dating anymore. I don't even know if they speak to each other. Facebook poking doesn't count. Everyone else could tell it was an unhealthy relationship that needed to end, but they just couldn't seem to do it. They wasted all that time and heartache for what?

Does your child know how to gently but directly turn down that next date? How to break up with integrity when that relationship is over? And how to manage through the inevitable hurt that will follow, without going back to that person for comfort or solace?

Put simply: You need to teach when to hold 'em, and when to fold 'em and walk away.

Chapter 13: Boundaries – They're Guardrails, Not a Straightjacket

When my husband first called my dad for permission to date me (as well as advice on how to do that. I played hard to get, to say the least), my dad immediately asked if we had discussed physical and emotional guardrails for our relationship. My husband confidently replied that we had, at which point he probably thought he had passed the test. My dad followed up with a request for a copy of that list. If there was any ambiguity about how we would be conducting our relationship, it was instantly cleared up. My husband faxed him the list the next day, with a very clear disclaimer that just because it was on the list did not mean that we had necessarily done it.*

* I came across that list the other day and I about died at what we wrote and sent. I don't even want to imagine my poor father's reaction as he read it. It was on the list to make sure we *didn't* do it!

Over the course of our relationship, until the day I walked down the aisle, my dad would regularly ask me how we were doing, specifically praying and encouraging us to hold to the guardrails that we had set. Nothing like your dad asking if you had kept your clothes on to make you hold the line! He wasn't all Napoleon Bonaparte about it. He was doing us a favor by helping us hold to our own commitment to honor one another and to maintain a high standard of purity until the day we became husband and wife.

What would be the point of me telling kids that they have it in them to wait for and expect more out of sex, if I couldn't do it myself? I'm a lot of things, but being a hypocrite is (hopefully) not one of them. We weren't perfect, but when we might have been tempted to go further than originally intended, we went back to the guardrails previously agreed upon, avoiding decisions that we would have regretted and even could have destroyed the relationship.

My dad's request for the list was exactly what I expected from him (Did I mention I was 23 years old AND living two states away? My dad=fearless. And awesome). I would have been surprised if he *hadn't* asked. Emotional and physical guardrails were always an important and continual part of our discussions about relationships, even before I was old enough to be dating. My dad knew that all the knowledge in the world about STDs, teen pregnancy, the complexity of my reproductive system, the sacredness of marriage, emotional bonds of sex, etc, etc, *might* not be enough to stop me if I got to that point where clothes started coming off, with hormones at full steam, and a cute boy making convincing professions of love. He knew I would need some practical tools to keep me from finding myself in that situation in the first place, or if I did, how to get out.

Most teens I speak with understand that sex is special, they want to save it, and may have even thought through *why* they're waiting. Sixty-one percent of teens want to be virgins when they get married.[43] Yet by the time they turn 19, seven out of ten male and female teens will have had sex.[44]

When people cross their personal line of waiting to have sex, it's rarely because they wake up one morning and joyfully proclaim, "Today, I'm going to compromise all the way and be swept asunder by passion. Damn the consequences!" No. They begin to justify small compromises that in themselves aren't much, but when added up together, undermine their decision to save sex for marriage. For many, it becomes a fairly passive decision, something that "just sort of happened."

Question: What do you think is the most common context for teens having sex?

A. After Prom, in a hotel room or at a co-ed sleepover.

B. A romantic, thoroughly planned evening.

C. At home, late at night while their parents sleep.

D. During a party, possibly while under the influence of alcohol.

If you picked C, you would be correct. In *Forbidden Fruit*, author Mark Regnerus found that the most common context for teens having sex was at home, late at night *while their parents slept.* Even the risk that mom or dad might walk in on them was not enough to change their mind or put the brakes on what was happening.* I had a student tell me how her boyfriend had started to unbutton her pants while they were kissing, even though her parents were right in the next room, very much awake. I'm happy to report that she promptly pushed him off, making it clear that when she said boundaries, she meant it. She must have had a really good Relationship Speaker come to her school (wink).

*A side question is why would you as a parent go to bed when your son or daughter has a date over?? That's like leaving the gas on with an open flame nearby and not expecting your house to blow up. You're asking for trouble and not doing your child any favors.

As a parent, you will not always be there when your child is alone with the opposite sex – unless you're planning on moving into their college dorm. And even that isn't a guarantee. Better to give them the tools they will need to succeed in that moment, when it comes, so you can keep sleeping soundly. College parties are way overrated these days anyway.

What is in a name?

You have probably heard emotional and physical parameters in a relationship referred to as, "Boundaries." Here's the problem I have found while speaking to teens; that word has a negative connotation in most of their minds, as though boundaries are a straightjacket they're forced to wear until someday they break free and get married. Rather than understanding that those boundaries are there to help, teens see them only as a hindrance to fun and enjoying life.

When you drive up a canyon road, there running alongside the edge are guardrails. Why? To show you how far you can go and still be safe. If you were to cross the guardrail, your risk of injury increases, particularly if it's a steep drop-off to a valley below. No one in their right mind sees those guardrails and angrily crashes into them, declaring, "You're holding be back from having so much FUN!"

That is why we're renaming boundaries to guardrails. They are there to help your child understand how far they can go physically and emotionally and still be safe. Rather than holding them back from enjoying life, they're actually optimizing their chances of freedom, health, and happiness. By explaining it this way to our children, they'll come to see them as a positive, rather than a negative, and be more motivated to uphold those guardrails on their own because they understand *why* they're in place.

On the next page is a little form created to help you begin to define the guardrails you deem appropriate for your son or daughter's relationships. This builds on that outrageously fun activity you did a few pages back, where you defined what you thought about sex, when it was appropriate for your child, and what the ideal scenario would be for that. See, I had a point. For those of you that skipped it, go back and do it!

Talk these over with your spouse or your child's other parent(s) so you can agree on what the appropriate guardrails are for your son or daughter. As with any aspect of parenting, a united front is key.

Your Preferred Guardrails

Add to this list as you desire. This is just to get the train moving.

1. At what age is your son or daughter permitted to group date?
2. One-on-one dates?

3. At what point in the relationship would you like to meet the boyfriend/girlfriend?

i.e. when they first pick them up for a date or after three dates?

4. Before your son or daughter head out on a date, which of the following are required?

- Sharing with you the plan or schedule
- Knowing what time the date will be over and what time you can expect them to come home
- Contact information
- Other:

5. If the date is going over to the opposite sex's home:

- Will the parents be home?
- Have you met the parents?
- Do they hold similar values in this area and hold to similar boundaries for their child?

6. Is there a curfew? What is the protocol if your child is going to be late?

7. Will you be waiting up for them to come home from a date or do they need to wake you when they get home?

8. What are appropriate boundaries if your son or daughter is with their date at your home or the dates?

- Parents must be home
- Lights must remain on when watching a movie
- If hanging out in a bedroom, door must be kept open
- Other:

9. Which of the following scenarios do you think are appropriate and at what point in the relationship?

- Alone in a bedroom
- Sleeping over
- Hand Holding
- Kissing
- Heavy Making Out
- Cuddling
- Excessive Public Displays of Affection
- Oral Sex
- Fondling/Hands under shirts & down pants
- Sexual intercourse
- Other:

This is not a dictatorship.

With a clear understanding of where you stand on the issue and the boundaries you prefer, ask your teen what they think. Exchange ideas on what each of you consider appropriate, then come up with a list that you have both agreed on. You'll notice there was a lot of team work/partner/togetherness in those last two sentences. No "I" in Team here. This actually works to your benefit however. Since your teens helped define said boundaries, they'll have a greater sense of ownership. Much more fun than simply implementing martial law and bracing for the revolt.

In the chapter title, I referred to boundaries as guardrails, rather than straight jackets. The idea of boundaries can conjure up images of being boxed in, cut off from enjoying the good life and having any fun. But guardrails on a mountain road are there to provide protection, demarking the point between what is safe and what is potential danger. No sane driver sees them as restrictive, holding them back from being able to really enjoy life by careening over the edge. That is the imagery we need to use when talking to our teens, the distinction they need to understand. Whether you call them boundaries or guardrails, they are there to help your son or daughter know how far they can go and still be safe, and at what point do they cross into a potentially dangerous area.

Some questions to get the conversation going:

- What are responsible and safe guardrails?

- How far are you willing to go on a first date? Third date? Once you become exclusive with someone?

- How serious do you think relationships should get in high school?

- What do they think about kissing? Oral sex?

- Are there ever circumstances where they think they could be tempted to compromise?

(i.e. making-out in the dark or while laying down, if they've been drinking, after a certain time of night.)

- How do you think you would feel if you went 'this far' with your date? This far? Could it affect your reputation? Your self-esteem?

- What are some potential consequences that could happen from going too far physically? Emotionally?

- What are emotional guardrails that should then be put in place? Physical guardrails?

Some Examples of Physical & Emotional Guardrails

- Avoiding situations where there are no adults present.
- Not pouring your heart out on the first date.
- Becoming friends first before dating.
- Having a clear idea of sexual boundaries: what will best protect your body and your heart?
- Balance of time spent together and time spent with other friends, family, doing sports, schoolwork.
- Respecting that person's personal time.
- Paying attention to what your clothing says about how you view yourself and how you want others to view you. Our wardrobe can speak volumes about our expectations and boundaries without us ever opening our mouth.
- Clear plan for dates with a predetermined time to be home; curfew
- Going on "intentional" dates to see each other in various situations (i.e. going out with groups, double dates, volunteering together, picnics, concerts, etc.)
- Limiting the amount of time spent talking daily/weekly (via phone, email, text, Facebook, or in person)
- Group Dates

- Fighting fair
- Staying sober
- Pacing out how much your share

As you are discussing these guardrails, it is important to also talk about what happens if they find themselves having crossed them some day. When students write to tell me that it's too late for them because they've already made sexual choices they regret, my heart breaks for them. It is NEVER too late to go back, to begin again.

Our teens need to understand that when they make mistakes, when they cross their limits (Yes, when. Moments of weakness happen to the best of us. Don't forgot how persuasive hormones can be), it does not mean that guardrail no longer holds value, or is irrelevant. Some of your teens have already given or received oral sex, or may have already had sexual intercourse. They are wondering how to go back, whom they can turn to in order to deal with the pain and what this means going forward. Are they damaged goods? Does this mean they can't say no the next time someone asks them to go that far again?

Guardrailsare there to help your child navigate their way safely and successfully through relationships, like guardrails on a road. They are not there to be a set of rules or standards your child feels they have to live up to so that you will be proud of them and love them. You can have all the right intentions, but if your children feel your love for them is conditional, based only on how well they meet a certain set of expectations, or how good they appear to be, you will leave them feeling as though they are never enough, and drive them away.

HOW YOU DO IT

The quickest way for a parent to get a child's attention is to sit down and look comfortable.

Lane Olinghouse

Chapter 14: This is a Dialogue, Not a Monologue

I was on a radio show when a mother called in, clearly frustrated:

> *"It doesn't matter how much you teach them in terms of their integrity, their reputation, their character, being pure, keeping those boundaries. We can ... talk **TO** them over and over again about your reputation is how people see you...that you have to keep your boundaries true to your own purity and you can talk **TO** them about all these things but once they get to that school, or out with their friend, it seems to go with the wind."*

What stands out to you about her statements? All the times she emphasized talking TO her teens? You're so observant, well done.

Who likes being talked *to*? No one! Especially not teenagers. These talks on sex and relationships are not monologues to be delivered forcefully, albeit quickly. You'd be better off talking to the wall if this was the case. Besides, it would probably show more enthusiasm.

It is a conversation, a dialogue, an exchange of words. Which takes some of the pressure off of you! You are not expected to deliver a prepared five-point presentation. I'd like to kindly request that you never ever do that. Do not, do not, do not talk TO your child. That will only reaffirm their belief that you are out of touch and not someone to come to with their questions. Talk WITH them. You might start the conversation, hear their response, and so forth. Sort of like you do with other people that you respect and admire. Or you'll first say what boundaries you find appropriate, and then they may offer a rebuttal. Yelling or pained shrieks count as a response, at least in the beginning.

One effortless, unexpected, and minimally painful way to begin this dialogue is by using the world in which your child is already submersed.

As much as we like to blame the media for promoting messages of sex and sexuality that may not align with what you as parents believe, it wouldn't hurt to send the media and it's "subjects" a thank you card now and again. Why? Because of all the Kim Kardashian, Paris Hilton sex-tape-celebrities that regularly invade your home? Or because of content masterpieces like Jersey Shore, Gossip Girl, Pretty Little Liars and Glee? Hardly. But you *can* thank them for the jackpot of conversation starters with which they provide you.

Last year, a whopping 76% of teens that were surveyed about teen pregnancy said that what they see on TV about sex, relationship and love is a great way to start conversations on these topics.[45] That is some serious insider information you just received!

If your son or daughter loves a certain TV show, sit down and watch it with them. Use what is brought up in the episode as a segue into these conversation. If they *don't* want you to watch with them, this is also a perfect opportunity to ask what about the show makes them uncomfortable for you to be around. Movies, advertisements, news articles, magazines, or even your friend's pregnancy can all provide teachable moments. You are simply looking for opportunities within their world, to bring up the topic and to focus their thoughts on the messages around them to which they may be oblivious. In the process, you're teaching them to become media literate – able to interpret the messages promoted and the impact they have on their life and culture at large. Plant multiple seeds of information that get lodged into different corners of their brain, coming at the issue from every angle. You never know which seed will be the very thing that saves them that next time they're out with their friends and tempted to do something risky.

Keep an ear out for what your child is saying on the phone when they talk to their friends, or conversations between your kids. You don't need to go so far as hiding a baby monitor under their bed. Once you start actively tuning in to their conversations, you'll be surprised how openly your kids talk to their friends even though you're right there in the next room. How and what they talk about will give you a clue as to where they are at in their learning and curiosity.

Gently and in a non-confrontational way, bring up what you heard them discussing, asking what they think about the issue, if they have questions, or if their friends are dealing with this. It is critical that when bringing up something you overheard, that you do so in a way that does not put them on the defensive or make them feel unsafe or distrustful. The last thing you need is to confirm your child's suspicions that you have nothing better to do than eavesdrop on them.

Wrong: "I heard you talking to Tommy about a girl at school that you're interested in. You better be careful. Do you know what kind of girl she is? Does she know that sex could get her pregnant and that you're not that kind of guy?! I mean, that would be the end of my Harvard dreams for you!!"

Right: "I couldn't help but overhear you talking to Tommy about a girl at school. Hope that was ok. Sounds like you're interested. Want to tell me about her? I'd love to hear, but completely understand if you're not ready to talk about it yet."

The only response you might get at first is a skeptical look to see if this is really happening, but continue to be persistent. How you initiate these first few conversations will set the tone for the talks you'll have down the road, and whether or not your son or daughter engages.

Encourage communication

It's not just enough to strategically make the most of easy introductions for nuggets of gold and well-placed questions. You also want your child to respond in those moments, or – fairy tale of fairy tales – to actually come to you on their own with a question, and to tell you about what is going on with their friends or even their own situation. Something that gives you a bit more insight beyond their Facebook Relationship Status of "It's Complicated." There's just one teeny tiny problem: Teenagers do not talk. At least not to parents. There's no end of conversations with their friends (as your cell phone bills prove). But for you, getting two words from them about their day is a superhuman feat. Even more so if you have boys.*

So what if you don't get a verbal waterfall from them the first time you venture into this barren wasteland? Do not give up! Like a lion pursuing a gazelle, you must be relentless. Pursue opportunities to talk, encourage communication, and emphasize that whenever your child is ready to talk, you're all ears. To hear anything. And no matter what they tell you, you are still going to love them unconditionally. Don't forget that you also need to do everything in your power to remain calm. By encouraging your teens to talk, you reinforce that you really are a safe place for them to open up.

How then do you create a safe place for them to let down their guard and talk about what is really on their heart?

One thing teenagers (and really, most of us) hate is being on the receiving end of a probing question that seems

* I know because I have 5 younger brothers.

just a little too personal. How would you feel if your mother asked you, "Have you ever had oral sex or thought about having it?" That's what I thought. But you need to bring it up, to educate on this oh-so-proper topic, so try a different approach. "I read that more teens are having oral sex because they think it's safer. What do you think of that? Think it's true?" Or, "Did you know that alcohol use by teens is associated with risky sexual behavior? Why do you think that is? What would you consider 'risky'?" This goes hand in hand with taking advantage of teachable moments. It is a great segue into making it more personal and more about them. You're not asking them to read to you from their diary – you are showing that you're aware of what might be going on in their world, and that it's not all that shocking to bring up these topics. Not to mention that the look of shock that will pass their face when you first utter those words will be priceless.

Tell them WHY

Rewind a few years to when your child was just beginning to explore the world around them. Aside from "no," what other favorite word of theirs almost drove you to a nervous breakdown?

"Why?"

Sometimes it was followed by a take-your-breath-away question, other times it was just left to dangle, daring you, goading you. At that age, they didn't quite understand how infuriating their merry-go-round of Why's could become. The magic pill in all of it was that they were still satisfied to believe that because mom and dad said so, it therefore was. Ah, what you wouldn't give to have that now. The dreaded "Why?" has come back, only this time with attitude, and the expectation of an actual explanation. "Because I said so," is not going to be good enough. At this point, that will be akin to throwing lighter fluid on a fire of teen frustration, angst, irritability, and emotional uncertainty.

Here's my million-dollar solution: when your teen asks 'Why?' tell them. Tell them your good reasons for not wanting them to be out past curfew, why you want to make sure that parents will actually be at the party, why you want to know what their plan is for the date, why you require they reply when you text late at night, or why ..... (insert your own). When they were young, they may not have been ready for all the reasons. They hadn't learned how creepy clowns really are or that some people aren't actually nice.

But now, with only a few months, or at best, years, before your child spreads their wings, it is your job to teach them about this wonderfully tragic, beautiful and frightening world and how to live in it without becoming destroyed by it.

Melodramatic? Me? No, it is the wisdom of being able to look back at life and see how much my parents taught me and how much heartache they saved me from as a result. I sometimes shudder to think who I might have become had I not had parents who were invested every step of the way and never stopped answering my "Why?" I didn't ask it to be difficult (at least not most of the time), but because I simply wanted to understand their reasoning behind a particular decision. Only then could I trust that when they said yes or no, it was because they really had thought through what could happen and that they had my best interest in mind. They weren't simply thinking of themselves or how my actions might reflect on them, or because they had this incredible need to be in control; it is because they loved me and wanted the very best for me. Bonus was that it also taught me how to build proper trust with my husband. So consider it an investment in your child's future relationships. Their spouse will thank you someday. Even if they don't quite know why.

I know that taking the time to explain "Why?" every time, is going to wear on you, that your nerves are going to become frayed. Especially when they still roll their eyes, stomp off to their room in a huff, and text their friends about how miserable you're making their life. I know you want only the best for your child. But it's not me you have to convince. It's your son or daughter. When they're asking why, they're really testing you to see what your motivation is: their well-being or your need to be in control? They *will* think about what you had to say, and might even secretly be grateful. Just because you're the parent doesn't mean you have to be the one in the hot seat the whole time. Feel free to give them a taste of their own medicine (although without the attitude). Be the better (wo)man who at all times turns the question around and asks, "Why?"

"Why do you want to go out that late?"
"Why don't you want me to talk with the parents?"
"Why do you think I'm being too hard on you?"
"What would you think is more reasonable?"

You are still the parent, you still have the final say, but it will go a long way in opening communication and strengthening trust if you are willing and able to verbalize your why.

Chapter 15: The Art of Listening...and Not Having a Heart Attack About What You Hear

We all have someone in our life (or maybe more than one) who is a terrible listener. You can see the wheels turning in their head as they form their next sentence, just waiting for you to pause long enough for them to jump back in. One breath, and you lose your chance to speak again for the next five minutes. Maybe they don't even let you finish, cutting in with their well-meaning advice or some experience from their own life that they think is JUST like what you were talking about. Except it's not, at all. Or they continually pepper you with questions before you have even had a chance to finish what you are saying. They might say they're hearing you, but are they really *listening*?

As parents, you have more perspective, life experience, knowledge and wisdom than your teens, which in time, they will need to hear. Add to that all the new information you've picked up from these gold trimmed pages and it can be tempting to want to share everything with your teen the moment they first show any sign of life. This might be your only shot! Resist. Sit on your hands if necessary (I find it extremely difficult to talk if I can't use my hands). Because if you overwhelm, overreact, or over-share, you probably won't get a second chance.

Once you get your child to open up, you'll want to hear what they have to say, and more importantly, what they are *not* saying, but subtly hinting at. How you listen will determine whether this is a one-time anomaly or the beginning of ongoing conversations. If you want them to actually hear what you will eventually say, to internalize and make life decisions with your words in mind, then you will have to earn that right.

Gone are the days when your child hung on your every word, unquestionably following your direction and submitting to your guidance, when their incessant "Why?" wasn't them purposely trying to get under your skin. Gone are the days when you were the center of their world, infallible, and all knowing. Now, 98% of what you say is met with disdain, rolled eyes, frustration, and attitude. And that is *if* you can get them to take their headphones off and stay in the room long enough for you to finish your sentence. If it's any consolation, my parents suddenly became much smarter, wiser, and even likable when I hit college. I'm not making any promises here, but there's most likely a light at the end of this very dark tunnel.

But you can't wait until then!

If you don't start properly talking about sex until they've moved out of the house, it will be too late.

Even if your kids are respectful and actually seem to listen to what you have to say, is it relevant to what they are facing, to the temptations and struggles they face daily? Do you know what is actually going on inside their heart and head? The 'good' kids are just as tempted by sex and drinking as those we label the 'rebel' or 'troubled' teen. There is incredible pressure on kids today to live up to a certain standard, and many look for release from that pressure in unhealthy ways.

Regardless of how good you think your kids are, how safe their behavior is, or how much you think this book doesn't apply to you, you will waste you breath talking to them if you first do not *listen.* Not just being in the room or car when your teen is talking, but actually putting down the cell phone, turning away from the computer, shutting off the TV and really listening to what your teen has to say.

The following four tips may seem deceptively simple, but take the time to really master them. It will make a huge impact towards this becoming a two-way conversation, rather than a one-way street with you in the driver's seat.

1. Be a good listener

That means you stop talking. Did I already say that? Then maybe it's important. As your mother says, you have two ears and one mouth. When your child starts opening up, you might start acting like a brand new puppy tripping all over yourself with excitement to share, crashing right into what your child is saying. We don't *mean* to interrupt. We just so desperately want to share some very important information for that very thing they're talking about *right now*, that if we don't say it, they'll move on and the moment will be lost! Hey, calm down. It's actually more important to get to hear what your son or daughter has to say than to make sure your point is made. Priceless really.

Do NOT interrupt once your child opens up. And do not be mentally forming your response, waiting for them to take a breath and allow you to jump in. Teens have a BS radar like no one else, and can tell in a split second if you're not actually engaged. This is a big risk for them to open up to you, and if they get the slightest sense that you are not listening, that what they have to say is not all that important, their insecurities and sense of vulnerability will kick into high gear, shutting everything down and throwing those walls back up.

As they are talking, listen for what is not being said, for what they're really asking, but are too afraid to verbalize. When they finish, whether it was two sentences or a deluge for ten minutes, confirm what you hear with your child by restating it back to them. If this seems like elementary listening skills, that's because it is! I am coming to you as a peer mediator, certified in the 5th grade. So clearly I know what I am talking about. It was drilled into our heads that part of mediation is to have each side repeat back what they heard before speaking their piece. I thought it was the cheesiest thing. Reading that again, it still sounds cheesy. But here's the amazing thing. It actually works! Why? Because every person, regardless of age, status, race, blah, blah, blah, wants to know that they are being heard, that when they share their feelings, thoughts and opinions, it matters. Those things are an extension of who they are, and they want to know that who they are matters.

Think about how much confusion could be avoided in conversations if we made sure to first understand what the other person is saying. It is amazing how often we thought we heard correctly, only to find we were way off course.

Stop talking. Listen. And make sure you are hearing what their heart, their face and their eyes are saying when they share those words.

2. Address the topic at hand....but do not over-educate

Part of the reason you want to clarify what you're hearing is to save yourself from stepping right off the cliff. On the one hand, it can be tempting when your child asks a question to want to cram as much in your answer as time will allow, touching on everything that might remotely someday kind of sort of relate in someway, eventually. If this is your only opportunity to speak with your child, you have to make the most of it, right? But in doing so, you might actually over answer the question, giving your child more information than they were looking for, or is appropriate at their age.

For instance, if your seven year old comes home from school asking about oral sex, you launching into a detailed explanation of the mechanics, the risk of STDs or whether or not you think it's appropriate for them to do some day in the future is surely going to create more questions and confusion than your child initially started out with. Not to mention leave you scrambling to climb back up the cliff off of which you just fell. Take a moment to register your shock internally (more on that below), then ask some questions to feel out what they are really asking, and why, before you respond. Do they want to know because they heard someone talking about it? Did they see something? Or are they really asking something completely different and they have simply used the wrong words? Children mature physically and emotionally at different paces, so what might be necessary to discuss with one may be too much information, and even inappropriate, for another.

If it is your teenager, over-answering the question can risk coming off like lecturing, as though you're using every chance you can get to drive your point home, whether or not it actually applies. Remember, the point is *not* to have "The Talk." You want lots of opportunities to share new information, restate what has already been said, and approach the issue from different angles. It's like when you're reeling in a big catch....you do it slowly, a little at a time. There's no rush, and moving too fast will scare it off. Okay, it's a terrible analogy because you should not see your kid as a prize catch that you're slowly pulling in to slaughter. You get the point. Besides, what's a book without a fishing analogy?

3. Do not jump to conclusions

As you begin to create a safe environment for your child and foster open communication on sex, you will undoubtedly get a question that will register a slight heart palpitation. Internally, you are allowed to register shock. Feel free to be appalled about what you are hearing, to fill your spouse or friend in later at what you actually had to answer. But DO NOT let it register on your face or in your body language. Your child is gauging whether or not they can really come to you with questions, *any* questions. Sometimes they may ask something for the sheer shock value, other times because they genuinely want to know and still see you as the best source. If your son or daughter is willing to ask the shocking questions, consider yourself privileged and having done a great job in establishing trust. Every time I get a question that cuts my breath short, I remind myself that it's really a teen's highest compliment. They find me safe, informed, and even cool enough to ask what they're really thinking, but too afraid to utter to most anyone else. I have also developed a very good poker face.

The issue is not whether your kid has questions (for the zillionth time, they do!) but whether or not they feel comfortable bringing them to you. And when they do and they finally stop talking and look to you with those big Disney eyes full of curiosity, you *still* don't get to jump in like the Grand Coulee Dam just broke.

4. Ask Permission to Speak

Ask your son or daughter if they would like to hear your thoughts and opinions. My money says this will definitely shock them. Some of you are staring at me in disbelief, wondering why you even spent those measly few dollars on this lousy book. ASK if you can give your advice? Why, you're the parent and therefore have a right, even an obligation, to give your opinion! Technically, yes. But what is our objective here, Solider? To establish trust, to open the doors for further communication, to help them feel safe and comfortable. And to give your words a better chance at actually being heard, and maybe, just maybe, making a difference.

By asking their permission to share rather than simply telling them, you affirm that what they had to say was important and this really is a dialogue, not just another ad hoc lecture for you to display your wealth of knowledge. If they say yes, it means your teens will actually be *wanting* to hear what you have to say, and asking for your advice. Then all of your hard learned wisdom will finally be put to good use! And if they say no, they don't want to hear your thoughts, then respectfully reaffirm that you are glad they opened up to you and are there if they have any other questions or want to talk further. And leave it at that.

There will be a time when they'll want to hear what you have to say. If you can earn their trust in this moment, you have a much better chance of them actually following your good advice. But this is a marathon, not a sprint. Some miles will be a breeze, while others will feel like a straight up-hill climb, requiring everything in you to keep pushing forward. That's why it's important to know why you're doing this and perhaps have that written out somewhere to remind you in those moments that seem especially difficult. It is worth it. Really. Your child will thank you someday for having taken the time to listen and show them you really did care about what *they* had to say, even more than you did about what *you* had to say.

Chapter 16: Adopt the Boy Scout Motto, "Be Prepared!"

"Does anal sex feel good?"

"I was with a girl I just met who had me lick Nerds Candy off of her butt......could I be at risk for anything?"

"How do I tell someone I'm having sex with that I want to stop?"

"Is masturbation wrong? What about dry humping?"

"What is Blue Waffle?"*

"If both the guy and the girl use condoms, does that make it safer?"

* "Blue Waffle" is slang for a grossly infected vagina. If you were to look it up online, you would find that...it's a hoax. Sure, there is a disturbingly doctored up picture that looks like the inside of a very rotten oyster. What you'll also find is that it links to pornography. And all it takes is one look at porn for someone to get hooked. Which goes back to why you need to talk about it. This is what our teens are encountering when they innocently look up something they've heard in the halls of school.

"Is it normal to look at porn six times a day?"

"Can I get pregnant from giving a guy oral? Are you *sure*?"

Some of you, right now, may be particularly shocked and appalled that I would write these questions in this book. "How crass and unnecessary," you're thinking.

I did not make these questions up to make sure that you're still awake, nor did I put them in for cheap shock value. Those are questions I've received from 13 to 16 year olds, *many of them in private, religious schools.* Not in the low-income schools, or simply in 'other' neighborhoods that are worlds apart from yours.

If it were one kid, it would be a joke. Two kids, idle curiosity. When it's handfuls of kids asking the same questions, you quickly realize this is where teens "are at". These are the issues they are dealing with on a regular basis and what they wonder about, from Beverly Hills to Compton, the Hamptons to Harlem. If we want to be able to meet our kids on these issues, we must stop trying to sugar coat or deny the reality of the world in which they are growing-up. It's shocking, yes. But it is your teen's world, and one they desperately need you to enter into, in order to help them navigate it properly. For you to be able to confidently have conversations with your teens, you need to be educated. Part of the awkwardness surrounding sexuality is that we feel ill equipped to answer anything beyond the most basic questions. And we are even unsure how to navigate these questions! How can you expect to instruct your child, to be able to give reason and truth, without at least a base knowledge of the issues they are encountering on a daily basis? It is not enough to simply give our kids broad general statements about sex and hope and believe they will then commit to a life of sexual integrity. You have to give them something to really sink their teeth into, something concrete they can hold on to that speaks directly to where "they're at," to the questions, fears and curiosities they have. The high moral platitudes you generously dish out will be wasted.

Equip them, empower them with truth, with science, with facts, with knowledge, and *then* you can generously dish out your moral platitudes. You information and suggestions might go down a bit easier when they know you first care about their questions. Which, of course, requires listening. Yes, there it is again. As a parent, you need to become a student of your teen's world.

At the back of this book, I have compiled a list of web sites and books that I can confidently recommend to you as useful, informative resources. I weeded through some pretty terrible books and cringe-worthy websites to find those that maximize the information in the limited time you have. In other words, I dealt with the less than stellar resources out there so you wouldn't have to waste your time. You're welcome. Feel free to thank me in the form of Starbucks cards or cash.

You can find these and other books at libraries and bookstores. If you're married, make it a date and wander through until you find books that fit where your child is in their development, as well as what may appeal to them. Different books will be appropriate at different times, so go ahead and start hoarding for the years ahead. The changes will come sooner than you expect.

The websites I've listed have a wealth of information, from basic fact sheets, to extensive reports on teen pregnancy rates, abortion rates, condom use & effectiveness, STD trends, thoughts on teen sex from teens, from parents, what other parents are doing to talk to their teens, how the media influences teens, or how teen consumer trends influence the media. That should be more than enough to quell even the most inquisitive kid's questions.

Some have newsletters that you can sign up for to stay regularly updated on the changing terrain of teen sexuality. Read the articles and get a grasp of some of the information you can then pass on to your child. Check out some of the other sites that I've listed, to see what your teens may be looking at. These are the sites that are touting themselves as the experts to teens, and the source for their questions. This will help with the terminology, as well as giving you an eye-opening experience about what your teens are being taught by the world (in case you haven't owned a TV in five years or been outside in six months). And if everything I have said to this point has not been enough to motivate you to begin to talk about this, then these sites should do the trick. Your silence allows them to step in and be the educators of your children. Do you like what they're teaching?

Talk to other parents to find out how they are talking to their kids: what they have found that works and what has not worked (Hint: being in a locked car on a three hour road trip is a sure way to get yourself tuned out. And drive your child insane). You will find that you are not the only one with questions (you're normal!) and together, you can begin to effectively equip all of your kids. It will also ensure that when your kids go to someone else's home, you have peace of mind that the same messages, boundaries, and standards will be upheld. If you're going to do all this hard work, to actually talk about these things with your child, the last thing you want is to be undermined when he goes to Jimmy's house. It takes a village to raise a child. Or something like that.

Find educators that do this for a living. I have the luxury of spending hours a day educating myself on this, staying abreast of the latest information, articles, and trends, as well as interacting with thousands of teens. Individuals like myself can save you hours of time and help you address the specific questions. You do not have to read every book, article or report. Nor do you have the time! You're busy with jobs, the responsibility of a family, and trying to keep your sanity in a household of teen hormones. You need the quick and dirty version of what is relevant and effective; the Cliff Notes of teens, sex, and relationships in the 21st Century. Religious leaders and workers, be they pastors, priests, youth leaders, rabbis, etc, are also a great source, both for getting a pulse on what is going on amongst teens, as well as how to respond in ways that are consistent with your faith.

So you do all this research, start reading books, feel more knowledgeable about sex than you have ever been (aside from personal experience)...and your child asks a question that stumps you. Foul! Roughing the Ref. They can't do that...can they? They can and they do. It still happens to me! No matter how much preparation and research you may do, your child will manage to come up with that one question you have not yet thought through. Being prepared does not guarantee you'll know everything. When have you *ever* known everything, especially when it pertains to your kids? Don't worry, your secret is safe with me.

When the air gets sucked from the room you're in, you have two ways to respond:

1. Give the Oscar performance of a lifetime, acting the part of the well-informed parent who really hasn't a clue in heaven.

2. Admit that you don't know the answer and suggest that you try to find it *together*, whether on-line or in books.

The answer should be pretty obvious but for those of you a little slow on the uptake, here's a clue:

Scenario #1:

Your child quickly realizes you do not actually know the answer, but that you are trying to play the all-knowing-parent. Teens have a built in Authenticity Meter (the politically correct name for a Bullsh... Detector but this book has a PG rating) when it comes to adults. Like wild animals, they can smell fear, *your* fear, and will go in for the kill. They actually expect you to know less than they do about these issues. Why teens think this is beyond me, since they wouldn't be alive if you didn't know a thing or two about this whole sex thing. Regardless, trying to cover your lack of knowledge just destroys your credibility, making you unapproachable and weak.

Scenario #2:

Your weakness is actually a strength! Admitting you don't always know the answer will do wonders in opening up the dialogue and building trust between you and your child. Not to burst your bubble, but they've probably figured out you don't know *everything*. Best to come clean with yourself as well. Showing this vulnerability also affords you a great opportunity to spend time together, teaching your child how to discern what sources are credible, and how to properly navigate the Internet on these issues. Opening the door for further conversations down the road is a win all around. And very freeing. Try it out, you'll see what I mean.

Turn Your Kid into MacGyver

I hate to be the bearer of bad news, but there will come a day when you're not going to be there with your child to help make sure they make the right decision. They'll be at someone else's house, there will be a persuasive guy or aggressive girl that hasn't yet heard about your child's boundaries, a party where parents are not present, or they'll head to college far enough away that you can't just stop by on your way home. Neither will they pick up every call or answer your incessant texts. I know, it's rough.

So what are you to do, other than place a tracker on their car, phone, and under their skin once they fall asleep? In addition to teaching about fun facts, boundaries, and brain chemicals, you will want to equip them with clear information to be resourceful with when they face a risky or tempting situation, and to be able to think a decision through before going ahead.

I just lost some of you. I can tell by the glazed over look you're giving me. Your child might be able to rattle back how many people get an STD each year, what the difference is between bacterial and viral, or why their brain is just as affected as their body during sex, and yet find themselves making some very different decisions in the heat of the moment.

Even as they begin to look more like adults, remember that they are still very much kids when it comes to their emotional and psychological development and are still in need of parents. They may look like an adult, but they cannot fully reason like one, may not be able to determine the potential consequences of their actions, and may be more prone to impulsivity. Not until your child reaches his mid-twenties will the part of his brain that controls "proper decision making" be physically mature.

To put it another way, their body is growing during their teen and young adult years, and so is the part of their brain that is responsible for being able to make "complex assessments about future consequences."[46] What seems obvious to you as a possible outcome of a situation is less so to your teen.

It's been so long since you went through puberty, you may have actually forgotten how crazy those first few years are with rampant hormones, physical and physiological changes happening at a frightening pace, and your whole world being one uncontrollable emotional roller coaster. We can forget how easy it is for reason to get kicked out of the party the minute that cute co-ed walks through the door.

Add that to the increased pressure from peers and culture to be sexually active, to experiment, and the all too common presence of alcohol at underage parties.

Is your child prepared?

Train them to see the connections between their actions and possible consequences *before* it happens, by discussing possible scenarios they will face, how they could avoid them and what to do if they find themselves stuck. Train your child to think proactively about making healthy decisions, discuss what the consequences could be of poor choices and whether or not that is something they would want to face. Your child will, at some point, face a sticky scenario or two. Make sure they do so with eyes wide open, and with all the tools at their disposal to come out of that situation on top.

Confession: my parents didn't do this with me as much as they probably should have. They are absolutely amazing and everyone who hears of them agrees that they're pretty much the best parents ever (you have a shot at second place) but I don't think they, or I, really had an idea of what I would encounter at college. High school was rather tame and while we expected college to be a different environment (the copious amounts of alcohol we saw in the dorms during the campus tour was a pretty good tip off), we really had no idea what I was in for.

It's a miracle that I survived college the way I did, due in large part to their prayers, and the great job they did raising a girl who actually likes being different and stubborn in her convictions. That doesn't mean I didn't have some moments that are less than stellar, or lessons learned the hard way. Thankfully, none of them left any permanent damage or life-altering scars (emotional or otherwise). Even though my parents may not have discussed all of the following scenarios that you should address with your child, they did do a great job of cultivating in me the ability to think through the potential consequences of a choice. Which means that as much as I'd like to pretend that certain instances were simply me being swept away in the moment, it was actually a very conscious decision to ignore the vocal Jiminy Cricket in my head.

Feel free to use and adapt the following scenarios as is appropriate for your child. Add from your own experience, what their peers have gone through, or what your own teens have brought up in conversation (such as that co-ed sleepover they want to go to next weekend).

- Why dinner or a movie might be a better date than just hanging out on the couch downstairs without adult supervision.

- What to do if they get to a party where there is drinking and no adult supervision. Or drinking, period. Some parents are actually crazy enough to buy the alcohol themselves for their underage kids and their friends. (Oh ooops, that's you?? Yeah, TERRIBLE idea. I shouldn't have to explain why).

- What should you do if you're at a party or on a date where you didn't drive and you feel uncomfortable? How would you get out of that situation?*

- What if you're at college and people are drinking, and offer you a drink? You're not going to be driving anywhere. So is there any harm in accepting? What about two drinks?

---

* In the USA and Canada, you can dial #TAXI (#8294) for a cab, any time, anywhere. I strongly suggest you have your child put that in their cell phone, just in case of an emergency.

- What if you're on a date with someone and they start trying to push certain boundaries? How might you respond?

While your child is still under your roof, one incredible Get Out Of Jail Free card is being able to use you as an excuse any time. If they are in a compromising situation, or asked to go out with someone they are uncomfortable with, it may be easiest for them save to face by blaming you.

Examples:
"Oh, I'd really love to go to that party, but my parents want me home. Some family thing. I know, what a buzz kill."

"A date Friday sounds great! But my dad has this rule that every guy meet him first, and that the guy have a plan for the night, with a clear time set for when I'll be home."

Their friends may not think you are very cool but, they will have just avoided a potentially tempting situation while still saving face. For those of you that are trying to be the coolest parents on the block, this may be a hard one for you. Your purpose isn't to win "Most Liked" parents of the high school. You are there to protect your child, even if that means you are seen as the bad guy. Interestingly enough, most other teens will probably respect the fact that, as a parent, you are setting boundaries and are involved, especially if their own parents are not. Even as they act frustrated, teens are secretly wanting someone to set boundaries, to define for them what is ok and what is not ok. Remember, they feel out of control, and by you providing some structure, you create a more stable, secure world around them.

I have found that those parents who try to be their child's best friend, by allowing anything and everything in an effort to avoid any conflict, are actually hurting their children. They are not fighting for them; they are not fighting at all. Their own kids are saying to me, "I wish mom would make me do my homework. I wish dad would care who my friends were, and tell me I had to be home at a certain time."

What your child decides to do in relationships and in the area of sexual activity are some of the most important decisions they will ever make. Give them every resource available to make wise choices and avoid potentially damaging situations by fighting for them against this world, even if it means you look less than cool, or have to drive across town to pick them up at midnight.

The Secret Sauce

Be nice to your children, for they will choose
your rest home.
Phyllis Diller

Chapter 17: Relating to the Hormonal, Unstable, Yet Lovable Creature in Your Home aka Your Child

We both know you love your child very much. Even if you don't really like them right now. Which is okay. At the very least, they'll get more tolerable once they move out of the house. But no matter how maddening and downright spiteful they may be at times, there's nothing they could do that would end or diminish that love. If you need a quick reminder, look at some of their baby pictures for a few minutes.

Your love for your child is not based on anything they will ever do, but on who they are. They're your kid. Whether by blood or legal rights doesn't matter. They are yours and that is enough.

Do they know that? On some level, they probably do. But do they *really* know that? Have they internalized that to the core of their being? Is that understanding of unconditional love woven into the fabric of their identity?

In today's competitive, performance-based world, your child desperately needs to know that you will never base their value and worth upon how well they perform, upon whether or not they meet your expectations or if they are successful in the world's eyes. For a child, there should never be the expectation to be 'good enough' in order to be loved. Being is enough.

This needs to be the message your child receives every day, before, during, and after your conversations about sex. No matter what decisions they make on when to have sex and whether or not they stumble in their pursuit of sexual integrity, they should have the reassurance that mom and dad are still going to love them as much as they ever did. It has never been about meeting a certain standard or projecting a certain image to the neighbors. It has always been about wanting the absolute best for them.

Even as you applaud and encourage when they give it their best and do well in life, let it always be against a backdrop of unconditional, unwavering love. Tell them often. But more importantly, *show* them often.

Show and Tell:

What stands out to me from my teenage years, in regards to how my parents handled the issues of sex, identity, and relationships, are not the conversations we had about sex and its harmful side effects, the boundaries we defined together, or the rules about dating. What has left the greatest impact is how they treated me, how they showed love both to me and to each other, and the effort they made to regularly reinforce how incredibly special I was. How my dad treated me set the bar for what I expected from any guy that wanted to date me. I'll never forget the time I was having a terrible day and got called down to the school office. Waiting for me was a beautiful red rose with a note from my dad, for no other reason than to just remind me how much he loved me and that he was proud of me. I spent the next 15 minutes bawling in the bathroom, overwhelmed by what an insightful and loving father I had. If my dad could treat me this well, then it was reasonable that any guy trying to impress me and win my heart should do as well or better!

Valentine's Day always brought flowers, or a card or two, a tradition that stopped only once I got married, at which point my husband got to pick up the baton. Each week, one of my brothers or I would get one-on-one breakfast with dad.

In today's fast-paced, high-cost world, I know it may not be realistic for there to be a parent there whenever the kids come home from school, or to have the flexibility to rearrange your work schedule around their school events. Every family is unique. Please don't beat yourself up.

What does matter is that your kids *see* that you love them, understand it, and experience it every day. How you do this is going to be different for every child.

Do you take time out of your day to communicate your love? Maybe it is as simple as a text message in the day to say "I love you" or "I'm proud of you." Maybe it means leaving work early to attend a football game or canceling that business trip this weekend to spend some quality time with your kids. Time that doesn't involve both of you on a cell phone or staring at the TV.

Find ways to spend time with them, to engage them in those things that interest *them*. Computers may be foreign to you, but your child could build one from scratch. The ballet puts you to sleep, but your daughter could eat, sleep, and breathe it. You love sports, but your son loves video games. Roughing it to you is a Motel 6, while your child's best day would be hiking, turning over rocks to find strange bugs, and spending a night under the stars. By entering their world, you show that you care about who they are, with all of their unique interests, talents, and personality quirks. You open up the door for communication and may find out things about your child you never knew. Spending this time together will speak volumes about your love without you ever having to say a word.

Some of you may need to downsize your standard of living, to cut back on your hours, to minimize how much time you or your spouse spend outside of the home on your individual activities, in order to make this happen. Too harsh? Then you might need to reevaluate your priorities. In a family with six kids, on one salary, we didn't have a ton of extras. But we had parents who were available and present. And a ton of fun being together as a family. We didn't need a bunch of 'stuff' to be happy. Given the choice, I'd do it the same way again.

You have a brief 18 years where you get to see your child every day. Eighteen years that you get to pour love, affirmation, and instruction into another human being in a way that you will not get with many other people. Even if they move home after college, the relationship will be drastically different. Your presence will speak volumes to your child about what is important to you (hint: them). By being involved in your child's life, you fill that longing they have for love and affection, and minimize the chances that they will go searching for it somewhere else.

Buying them the latest gadget or upgrade on their phone, because you feel guilty about not being around, does not count as you showing them love. Time, interest in who they are, and again, time, is what matters here.

If you are not in the habit of regularly hanging out with your kids, it may feel weird at first. But keep at it. Your child will notice that you are saying no to other things, to say yes to being with them. Trust me, it makes a difference. Then, when you do bring up more serious topics like sex and relationships, you'll already have built the trust in your relationship that assures your child that you're saying things they may not understand or agree with out of love, not out of a parental obligation to cover "The Talk."

There has never been any question for my five younger brothers and me that sexual integrity, and waiting until marriage, was and is, the best route for our physical, emotional, mental, and relational health. But that standard was couched in a deeply ingrained understanding of, and confidence in, our intrinsic value. It has been clearly shown and communicated to us that we deserve the best in relationships, that we deserve to know an individual truly loves us and cares about what is best for us. We were taught to be certain of their commitment before giving so intimately of ourselves. We learned that real love and healthy relationships require work and sacrifice and that sex is just a piece of the whole. Now that I'm happily married, I can't thank my parents enough for raising that bar and teaching us that we could wait for the best.

At the end of the day, it probably won't be a scary statistic about an STD that will keep your son or daughter from going too far. It will be that quiet confidence within them that reminds them that their body, their heart, and their future matter greatly, and should be treated as such.

Emphasize that you are there to fight FOR, not WITH your child

Depending on the time of day, your teen's current mood, the position of the sun, and the present situation, they may see you as either the British Allies or Nazi Germany (it's dramatic but then so is your child). You are the enemy standing in the way of their growing up, of their becoming an adult, you don't want them to have fun, and have forgotten what it's like to be a teenager. Of course, it's the very fact that you *do* remember what it's like that you set boundaries, make rules, and in general, are trying to protect them from making a stupid, life changing decision. Remember how you saw your parents when you were that age? Our teens are struggling to create their own identities and part of that process is to push back. They need to break down what they see as your beliefs and values and then re-build their own. And, as they struggle with feeling out of control, confused and emotional, they are testing you to see if you will be the safe, stable, and dependable one in their world.*

In explaining your "Why," emphasize repeatedly that you're trying to fight *for* them, not *with* them. To fight for their safety, for their well-being, for the chance to have a future full of possibilities, for their success in school, relationships, and life. Your "rules" about what age they can start dating, requiring the guy to meet you

* Shanti Feldhahn and Lisa Rice have written a great book on this, surveying hundreds of teens to give parents a look into your child's thinking and perspectives. For Parents Only is on the list of resources in the back of this book that I highly recommend taking a look at.

(if you have a daughter, that better be on your list), wanting to know the plan for the date, setting boundaries, restricting certain activities, or asking numerous questions are part of your way of protecting. Be sure to simultaneously communicate that you are doing so because you love them and want to help them make the best possible decisions, not because you get some sort of sick pleasure from locking horns with them. Your son or daughter needs to see you as being part of their team, one of the few people in their life who will always be in their corner.

There will be times you'll be required to fight with them in order to fight *for* them, a subtle but important difference. Keep that distinction in mind and remember too that you are dealing with an emotional, unsure, confused teenager. Don't take it personally, or lower yourself to their level (or rise, depending on how loud their voice gets). You need to be their rock and their calm – to keep them level when they feel very much out of control. And do us all a favor by avoiding that terrible line, "This hurts me more than you." It didn't work when we were spanked and it won't work now amidst the arguments, curfews, and groundings. Trust me.

Chapter 18: Take a Look in the Mirror

Your child will learn the most about relationships from watching *you*. Watching how you treat them, how you treat your spouse or significant other, and how you allow yourself to be treated. The great thing about this is that you began modeling this from...the moment they were born. Your kid is already 8 years old? Oh, well, hopefully the last 8 years have been full of you subconsciously modeling relational awesomeness. I didn't say perfection, just awesomeness. We can tell kids until we are blue in the face that a good relationship should have communication, should be one in which both people are encouraged to grow, should have mutual love and respect, and whatever other cliché statements you would like to throw their way, but what does respect *look* like? How can you tell when someone is making you a better person or killing you softly? What does it look like to be more in love 20 years later than you were the day you got married?

Webster's won't be of much help here. Children, teens and even young adults need to *see* this on a daily basis. Your relationships provide a front row seat for them to see the ins and outs, the work that goes into a relationship, what is acceptable and what is a deal breaker.

They will model their relationships based on what they see you do and how you treat your spouse and your children.

How was that for sobering? There is plenty of research that show women end up marrying men similar to their fathers. Even if their dad was a total deadbeat loser. It's what they know, what they think they deserve, and healthy or not, the prominent male figure in their life. But you don't need the stats and studies to know that. Look at real life. You'll see that I'm right.

Have you ever tried to look at your relationships from your child's perspective? What do you see? A relationship you want them to model to the last detail? Great, keep it up. For the other 98% of us who are honest enough to admit no relationship is perfect, how can we improve? What can we do better? Do you need to be quicker at apologizing? Could it be as simple as daily saying, "I love you," or planning a regular date night to show your spouse they matter? Do you serve and encourage on a regular basis or have you become a bit stuck in your own ways? How patient are you, really? Are you a 4th of July show just waiting to explode?

Don't get all huffy with me! I'm just asking the questions here. Yes, I'll admit I'm trying to prod you a bit and even get under your skin, if that's what it takes to make sure your child is getting the best.

What if you're married to someone who in no way wants to work with you on this, who is that deadbeat loser or absent parent? All is not lost. Your example, both in how you treat your spouse and how you treat your kids, will still speak volumes. Do not underestimate the influence that you have in your child's life. There may be other adults in their life as well who are providing a healthy example and whom you can point to as models worth following. This also applies if you a single parent.

When was the last time you took your own kid on a date? They could be 5 or 15 years old, but you should still take them out. How are they supposed to learn that the guy opens the door when you get out of the car or that a woman should not order the most expensive thing on the menu just because she can? More of this will be discussed in Dating Basics. If you want the best for your

kid, set the bar high for them by showing them what they deserve, by modeling it in your own relationships, and by daily affirming it in what you say.
Married, single or divorced, you have a responsibility to set an example. "Do as I say, not as a do," is a terrible way to parent. And a sure fire way to insure your child will do exactly as you do, not as you say.

You can emphasize sexual integrity, the importance of waiting, and the awesomeness of marriage until you are blue in the face but if you are modeling something very different with your own life, your words will fall on deaf ears. You need to show that you believe what you are asking of your children, that it really does make a difference physically and emotionally to save sex for marriage, and that it can be done.

If you are currently not living a life of sexual integrity, by sleeping around, cheating on your spouse, inviting boyfriends/girlfriends to stay the night or looking at pornography, you need to stop. Now. Get whatever help you need to set the necessary boundaries and accountability, but stop. Right now. Nothing else you do is going to matter if you are not, yourself, living a life worth modeling.

Chapter 19: The Almost End

A very wise man once told me, "Joanna, there are two kinds of hard: short term and long term. If you give in to whatever you desire and what feels good in the moment, then it will be easy for the time being, but the long term could be very painful. Or you can endure the struggle of saying no to being sexually active, of sacrificing what you may want at the time or what is easy in the moment, so that in the long run, there will be no risk of regret, of painful memories, broken dreams, or an STD. You'll be able to build a relationship on trust, communication, and a habit of practicing faithfulness. It is going to be hard either way. You have to pick which hard you want."

It is going to be difficult for our kids either way, whether they practice sexual integrity or choose to be sexually active. We shouldn't try to gloss over this, or be unrealistic in our projections. Sexual integrity is hard stuff; it is not popular (yet) and it will require a certain amount of sacrifice and self-control from your teen. As they live out their commitment, they need to be reminded that the good they are giving up in the moment is so they can enjoy the best in the future.

The same goes for you. It's going to be difficult whether you choose to talk to your child or keep silent. One will require effort, vulnerability and learning. It might bring tears, get messy, and involve your child yelling. The other will maintain the status quo and peace in your home for the time being, but leave you to watch your child make some painful and avoidable mistakes on their own.

For both you and your child, it will take resolve, day after day, through thousands of small decisions. Along the way, they will make mistakes. So will you. That's okay. It's only in trying, that you can actually fail. Or succeed.

I hope this book has inspired you to begin (or continue) these conversations, giving you hope that you *can* do this, and that you *need* to do this. More than anything, I hope you understand that we need to be talking about this in a radically new way.

Rather than trying to use scare tactics or focus on fear, let us speak of sex out of excitement for what it *could* be, painting a picture for our sons and daughters of a version of sex that is better than what the media or their friends can offer. Sex is a good thing. A great thing! And we want our young people excited for the day they will get to enjoy it with their whole person: mind, body, and soul.

This is it. The end. The part where we say our tearful goodbyes and go our separate ways. What a journey this has been. We've laughed, cried, argued, and endured so much together. You started this book skeptical (it's okay, I didn't take it personally) and now, you're almost excited to go and do this. Or at least that's what I'm going to keep telling myself.

If I keep going, I'll become a blubbering mess, and I won't have you see me like that. Get out there and make me proud.

If at some point in all your glorious parent-child merrymaking, you want to drop a line to tell me how much I changed your life for good, brought world peace, whatever...I'd love that!

Or if this all goes terribly wrong and you find yourself ready to commit capital murder, I guess you can write as well.

Cheers!

Joanna Hyatt

Www.joannahyatt.com

Twitter: @JoannaHyatt

Facebook: www.facebook.com/joannahyatt1

Email: Questions@joannahyatt.com

Cell: Dream on.

THE END. Really. Good-bye.

Resources

WEBSITES

1. Center for Disease Control: www.cdc.gov

2. Fight The New Drug-Educating on the Harmful Effects of Pornography: www.fightthenewdrug.org

3. Focus on the Family: www.focusonthefamily.com

4. Mayo Clinic: www.mayoclinic.com

5. Medical Institute for Sexual Health: www.medinstitute.org

6. Office of Women's Health, US Dep. Of Health and Human Services: www.womenshealth.gov

7. The National Campaign to Prevent Teen and Unplanned Pregnancy: www.thenationalcampaign.org

BOOKS

1. *A Chicken's Guide to Talking Turkey With Your Kids About Sex*, by Dr. Kevin Leman and Kathy Flores Bell.

2. *Cyber-Safe Kids, Cyber-Savvy Teens: Helping Young People Learn to Use the Internet Safely & Responsibly*, by Nancy E. Willard.

3. *For Parents Only: Getting Inside the Head of Your Kids*, by Shaunti Feldhahn and Lisa A. Rice.

4. *For Young Men Only: A Guy's Guide to the Alien Gender*, by Jeff Feldhahn and Eric Rice, with Shaunti Feldhahn.

5. *For Young Women Only: What You Need to Know About How Guys Think*, by Shaunti Feldhahn and Lisa A. Rice.

6. *Hooked: New Science on How Casual Sex is Affecting Our Children*, by Dr. Joe S. McIlhaney Jr, M.D. and Dr. Freda McKissic Bush, M.D.

7. *How to Talk With Your Kids About Sex*, by Dr. John T. Chirban.

8. *Preparing for Adolescence: How to Survive the Coming Years of Change*, by Dr. James Dobson, Ph.D.

9. *Strong Fathers, Strong Daughters: 10 Secrets Every Father Should Know*, by Meg Meeker.

10. *Questions Kids Ask about Sex: Honest Answers for Every Age*, edited by J. Thomas Fitch and Melissa R. Cox.

11. *Unhooked: How Young Pursue Sex, Delay Love, and Lose at Both*, by Laura Sessions Stepp.

12. *UnProtected*, by Miriam Grossman, M.D.

SITES TARGETED TOWARDS TEENS

Listing these sites does not constitute as my endorsement. There are aspects that I agree with and others that I do not.

This is for you, as a parent, to be aware of what is being promoted by mainstream sites commonly viewed by teenagers. Use these as educational aides, at your discretion.

goaskalice.columbia.edu

gurl.com

itsyoursexlife.com

scarleteen.com

sexetc.org

stayteen.org

yourrealitycheck.org

Notes

[1] Center for Disease Control. Available at http://www.cdc.gov/hiv/topics/surveillance/resources/slides/adolescents/slides/Adolescents.pdf. (accessed August 11, 2011).

[2] Megan K. Beckett, Marc N. Elliott, Steven Martino, David E. Kanouse, Rosalie Corona, David J. Klein, and Mark A. Schuster, "Timing of Parent and Child Communication About Sexuality Relative to Children's Sexual Behaviors," *Pediatrics*, 2009. Available at http://pediatrics.aappublications.org/content/early/2009/12/07/peds.2009-0806.citation (accessed September 11, 2012).

[3] "Revealed: Oral sex is 'bigger cause of throat cancer than tobacco,'" *The Daily Mail* (online), February 21, 2011. Available at http://www.dailymail.co.uk/health/article-1358845/Oral-sex-bigger-cause-throat-cancer-tobacco.html (accessed July 29, 2011).

[4] Dr. Andrew Lange, "How to Get a Sexually Transmitted Disease Without Having Sex," *The Huffington Post* (online), June 28, 2010. Available at http://www.huffingtonpost.com/dr-andrew-lange/stds-how-to-get-a-sexuall_b_607797.html (accessed September 19, 2012).

[5] "Scientific Evidence on Condom Effectiveness for Sexually Transmitted Disease (STD) Prevention," July 2001, The National Institute of Health and The National Institute of Allergy and Infectious Diseases. Available at http://www.niaid.nih.gov/about/organization/dmid/documents/condomreport.pdf, (accessed August 15, 2011).

[6] Albert, Bill. "With one Voice 102: America's Adults and Teens Sound Off About Teen Pregnancy: An Annual Survey," Washington, DC: National Campaign to Prevent Teen Pregnancy, 2010. Available at http://www.thenationalcampaign.org/resources/pdf/pubs/wov_2010.pdf (accessed November 24, 2012).

[7] Ibid.

[8] Ibid.

[9] The Parent Gap: Teen Pregnancy and Parental Influence, A National Survey 2003, The National Campaign to Prevent Teen Pregnancy.

[10] Mary V. Merrill, "Generation Y: The New Global Citizens," Merrill Associates, http://merrillassociates.com/topic/2004/06/generation-y-new-global-citizens/ (accessed November 30, 2011). Reprinted with permission.

[11] Yes, there's a source for that. After all this time together and still no trust.
"The Waiting Game: Chastity Before Marriage May Have It's Uses After All," *The Economist* (online), January 20, 2011. Available at
http://www.economist.com/node/17956905
(accessed December 17, 2012).

[12] Kathryn Kost and Stanley Henshaw, "U.S. Teenage Pregnancies, Births and Abortions, 2008: National Trends by Race and Ethnicity, 2012." Available at http://www.guttmacher.org/pubs/USTPtrends08.pdf, (accessed September 19, 2012).

[13] Ibid.

[14] "Facts on American Teen' Sexual and Reproductive Health, December 2011," Guttmacher Institute. Available at http://www.guttmacher.org/pubs/FB-ATSRH.html. (accessed December 29, 2011).

15 "Why It Matters: Teen Pregnancy, Poverty, and Income Disparity," The National Campaign to Prevent Teen Pregnancy, March 2010. Available at http://www.thenationalcampaign.org/why-it-matters/pdf/poverty.pdf (accessed October 31, 2012).

16 Kate Perper, M.P.P, Kristen Peterson, B.A, and Jennifer Manlove, Ph.D, "Diploma Attachment Among Teen Mothers," *Child Trends, Fact Sheet: Washington, DC* (January 2010). Available http://www.childtrends.org/files/child_trends-2010_01_22_FS_diplomaattainment.pdf. (accessed August 3, 2011).

17 "50-State and National Comparisons: Teen Pregnancy Rate," The National Campaign to Prevent Teen Pregnancy. Available at http://www.thenationalcampaign.org/state-data/state-comparisions.asp?ID=3&sID=18&sort=rank#table, (accessed September 12, 2011).

18 "Gonorrhea- CDC Fact Sheet," Center for Disease Control, U.S. Government. Available at http://www.cdc.gov/std/gonorrhea/stdfact-gonorrhea.htm, (accessed June 15, 2011).

19 "STD Awareness Release," Center for Disease Control, U.S. Government. Available at http://www.cdc.gov/media/subtopic/matte/pdf/STDAwarenesMatteRelease.pdf (accessed May 29, 2009).

20 "Herpes- CDC Fact Sheet," Center for Disease Control, U.S. Government. Available at http://www.cdc.gov/std/herpes/stdfact-herpes.htm, (accessed June 15, 2011).

21 "HPV- CDC Fact Sheet," Center for Disease Control, U.S. Government. Available at http://www.cdc.gov/hpv/WhatIsHPV.html (accessed November 16, 2012).

[22] Workshop Summary: Scientific Evidence on Condom Effectiveness for Sexually Transmitted Disease (STD) Prevention, July 2001, The National Institute of Health and The National Institute of Allergy and Infectious Diseases. Available at http://www.niaid.nih.gov/about/organization/dmid/documents/condomreport.pdf (accessed September 12, 2011).

[23] "STD- CDC Fact Sheet," Center for Disease Control, U.S. Government. Available at http://www.cdc.gov/std/hiv/STDFact-STD-HIV.htm (accessed September 12, 2011).

[24] "Scientific Evidence on Condom Effectiveness for Sexually Transmitted Disease (STD) Prevention," July 2001, The National Institute of Health and The National Institute of Allergy and Infectious Diseases. Available at http://www.niaid.nih.gov/about/organization/dmid/documents/condomreport.pdf, (accessed August 15, 2011).

[25] "Birth control methods fact sheet," U.S. Department of Health and Human Services, Office on Women's Health. November 2011. Available at http://womenshealth.gov/publications/our-publications/fact-sheet/birth-control-methods.cfm (accessed October 31, 2012).

[26] Ibid.

[27] "This is My Reality: The Price of Sex," The National Campaign to Prevent Teen Pregnancy, January 2004. Available at http://www.thenationalcampaign.org/resources/pdf/pubs/My_RealityFINAL.pdf (accessed October 31, 2012).

[28] Joe S. McIlhaney Jr, M.D., and Freda McKissic Bush, M.D., Hooked: New Science on How Casual Sex is Affecting Our Children, 2008.

[29] Ethan Kross, Marc G. Berman, Walter Mischel, Edward E. Smith and Tor D. Wager, "Social rejection shares somatosensory representations with physical pain," *Proceedings of the National Academy of Sciences*, April 12, 2011, Vol. 108, no. 15, pages 6270-6275.

[30] Albert, Bill. "With one Voice 102," 2010.

[31] Hooked, p. 20.

[32] Ibid.

[33] Anita Chandra, DrPH, Steven C. Martino, PhD, Rebecca L. Collins, PhD, Marc N. Elliott, PhD, Sandra H. Berry, MA, David E. Kanouse, PhD, Angela Miu, MS, "Does Watching Sex on Television Predict Teen Pregnancy? Findings from a National Longitudinal Survey of Youth," *Pediatrics* Vol. 122 No. 5 November 2008, pp. 1047-1054.

[34] Drew Zahn, "American teens: We want our virginity back," *WorldNet Daily* (online). Available at http://www.wnd.com/?pageId=263737#ixzz1GQGwFKPp (accessed March 2011).

[35] "Daily Media Use Among Children and Teens Up Dramatically from Five Years Ago," News Release, *Kaiser Family Foundation*, released Jan 20, 2010. Available at http://www.kff.org/entmedia/entmedia012010nr.cfm (accessed November 16, 2012).

[36] Amanda Lenhart, "Text, Cell Phones and Messaging: Text Messaging Becomes Centerpiece Communication," *Pew Research Center Publications*, April 20, 2010. Available at http://pewresearch.org/pubs/1572/teens-cell-phones-text-messages (accessed November 28, 2011).

[37] Kimberly J. Mitchell, David Finkelhor, Lisa M. Jones and Janis Wolak, "Prevalence and Characteristics of Youth Sexting: A National Study," *Pediatrics*; originally published online December 5, 2011; DOI: 10.1542/peds.2011-1730. Available at http://pediatrics.aappublications.org/content/early/2011/11/30/peds.2011-1730.abstract, (accessed November 16, 2012).

[38] "Sex and Tech: Results from a Survey of Teens and Young Adults," The National Campaign to Prevent Teen and Unplanned Pregnancy and *Cosmogirls.com*, 2008. Available at http://www.thenationalcampaign.org/sextech/PDF/SexTech_Summary.pdf (accessed January 10, 2013).

[39] "Pornography Statistics," Family Safe Media, Available at http://www.familysafemedia.com/pornography_statistics.html (accessed December 29, 2011).

[40] "Thirty percent of women, 70 percent of men confess to looking at online porn: study," *NYDaily News* (online) February 11, 2010. Available at http://articles.nydailynews.com/2010-02-11/entertainment/27056038_1_study-big-issue-problem (accessed November 16, 2012).

[41] "That's What He Said: What Guys Think About Sex, Love, Contraception, and Relationships," The National Campaign to Prevent Teen and Unplanned Pregnancy , 2010. Available at http://www.thenationalcampaign.org/resources/pdf/pubs/ThatsWhatHeSaid.pdf (accessed January 10, 2013).

[42] "Dating Abuse Statistics," The National Teen Dating Abuse Helpline. Available at http://www.loveisrespect.org/is-this-abuse/dating-violence-statistics (accessed December 29, 2011).

43 Drew Zahn, "American teens: We want our virginity back."

44 "Facts on American Teen' Sexual and Reproductive Health, December 2011," *Guttmacher Institute.*

45 Albert, Bill. "With one Voice 102," 2010.

46 Hooked, p. 50-51.